COMMUNITY-BASED PREVENTION

Reducing the Risk of Cancer and Chronic Disease

Community-Based Prevention

Reducing the Risk of Cancer and Chronic Disease

DAVID McLEAN, DAN WILLIAMS, SONIA LAMONT, AND HANS KRUEGER

UNIVERSITY OF TORONTO PRESS
Toronto Buffalo London

© University of Toronto Press 2013
Toronto Buffalo London
www.utppublishing.com
Printed in Canada

ISBN 978-1-4426-4530-1 (cloth)

Printed on acid-free, 100% post-consumer recycled paper with vegetable-based inks.

Library and Archives Canada Cataloguing in Publication

Community-based prevention : reducing the risk of cancer and chronic disease / David McLean ... [et al.].

Includes bibliographical references.
ISBN 978-1-4426-4530-1

1. Community health services. 2. Preventive health services. 3. Health promotion. 4. Cancer – Prevention. 5. Chronic diseases – Prevention. I. McLean, David, 1947–

RA644.5.C64 2013   362.12   C2012-907763-1

University of Toronto Press acknowledges the financial assistance to its publishing program of the Canada Council for the Arts and the Ontario Arts Council.

Canada Council   Conseil des Arts
for the Arts   du Canada

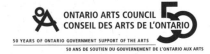

University of Toronto Press acknowledges the financial support of the Government of Canada through the Canada Book Fund for its publishing activities.

Contents

**PART B: OTHER MODELS OF COMMUNITY-BASED
PREVENTION EDUCATORS**

PART A

Purpose and Context

1 Introduction: Mastering the Surge in Chronic Diseases

Governments, communities, and health organizations around the world are struggling with the growing burden of chronic disease. This book offers important guidance on a promising response to one of the great public policy challenges of the present era.

It is not surprising that policy-makers are seeking ways to address such a severe test of their populations and economies. A sense of urgency may start with individual stories of suffering and loss, but it is quickly intensified by alarming information about chronic disease at an aggregate level.

Consider the following data:

- According to the Milken Institute, an independent economic think tank, the annual cost to the national economy in the United States of the seven most common chronic conditions (cancers, diabetes, hypertension, stroke, heart disease, pulmonary conditions, and mental disorders) is about $1.3 trillion, comprising $280 billion for treatment and $1 trillion in lost productivity in 2003.
- Based on current trends, the number of chronic cases in the United States would increase by 42% (to 231 million) by 2023 while the annual economic burden would jump from $1.3 trillion to $4.2 trillion.
- Globally, 60% of total deaths and 75% of disease burden (measured in disability-adjusted life-years) in those aged 30 years or over are due to chronic disease.

A Compelling Case for Prevention

Although the U.S. situation may be unique in some respects, the data are really just as dramatic in Canada, Europe, Australia, and, increasingly, countries in the developing world. Many national budgets are in danger of being swamped by rising chronic disease care costs, not to mention the impact in terms of suffering and poor quality of life. In light of these realities, the only long-term, sustainable hope for reducing mortality, morbidity, and costs due to chronic disease must be based on prevention efforts.

One advocacy group, Trust for America's Health, has concluded that an annual investment of $10 per person in proven community-based programs to increase physical activity, improve nutrition, and prevent smoking and other tobacco use in the United States could save that country more than $16 billion annually within 5 years. This is a return of over $5 for every $1 invested. A recent study in Manitoba by H. Krueger & Associates Inc. suggests a return on investment of 3:1 over a longer period. Although the cumulative gains are still small in terms of the overall cost of chronic disease, this sort of analysis does offer hope that the tide can at least begin to be turned.

Regional Realities and Responses

Leaders and the public alike respond to chronic disease statistics in different ways. National information can be helpful, but sometimes the overwhelming size of the numbers, combined with a lack of clarity about how they were calculated, can dampen the response of leaders. This is why it may be more beneficial to estimate chronic disease and/or chronic disease risk factor burden (using transparent and defensible methodologies) for smaller regions. It is valuable to break the total picture into smaller jurisdictions where policy interventions are still very pertinent.

For instance, the study in the Canadian province of Manitoba, which has a population of 1.25 million, calculated the 2008 economic burden of smoking, physical inactivity, and excess weight to be $1.62 billion ($492 million in direct health care costs and $1.12 billion in indirect costs related to productivity losses). If unchecked by successful prevention efforts, the annual burden would rise to $2.13 billion by 2026 – an overall increase of over 30% based simply on population growth and ageing.

Clearly, both the human and economic aggregate costs can be substantial, even for a relatively small population such as that in Manitoba. A case study focusing on current chronic disease prevention efforts in that province is presented later in the book. The sort of economic information summarized above is part of the core motivation for Manitoba leaders seeking to reduce the burden related to chronic disease risk factors. Even more compelling is a further analysis that concluded there would be substantial costs *avoided* if the prevalence of the key risk factors could be reduced just 1% to 2% each year.

This sort of "scaling" of information pertinent to prevention motivation and monitoring can continue, all the way to the regional health authority level and even municipalities and local health areas. Ultimately, whatever the size of the area and population being considered, it is likely that the sense of urgency about chronic disease will be consistent. The key question then is: *What to do about the challenge?*

Making Prevention a Priority

As already suggested, one response to the rapid rise in of chronic disease incidence and prevalence is expanding the capacity for treatment and care – but most would agree that there is a limit to continually meeting such an expectation within already burdened health budgets. Furthermore, the alternative approach of productivity gains and other system improvements eventually reaches a practical end-point.

Other responses entail what is sometimes known as primordial prevention, that is, avoiding exposure to risk factors in the first place, or primary prevention, reducing the duration of exposure in order to avoid the onset of disease – or at least at an early enough point that disease progression can be slowed or even reversed. These sorts of prevention efforts require long-term, concerted leadership.

It is important to recognize that the growing burden of chronic disease is a slow moving crisis – akin to a gradually rising flood. This is both the bad and good news of chronic disease epidemiology: while the situation is inexorably getting worse, the diseases in question, such as cancer, diabetes, and stroke, generally take a long time to develop in individuals. The same slow onset that allows medications, surgery, and other treatments to be effective secondary prevention measures also opens up the possibility of prevention earlier in the disease process. Risk factors can be reversed or, even better, avoided all together before chronic disease takes hold.

As the matter of "what to do" becomes clearer, the natural follow-up question is: *Who will lead the prevention effort?*

Who Will Stand in the Gap?

Reducing the level of, and damage from, a crisis such as a flood requires leadership and interventions at different levels. Large-scale, upstream projects such as dams and diversion channels can certainly be important; likewise, preparedness and focused responses at local levels downstream are often vital.

Fighting a flood provides an apt metaphor for prevention efforts related to physical activity, nutrition, tobacco use, etc. Policies (such as taxation strategies to reduce tobacco use) devised by higher levels of government need to be instituted; these are intended to influence either the whole population or at least at-risk subgroups of a substantial size. However, more localized responses are also very important. Broader policy requires input from leaders "on the ground" who gather information about the potential and actual effects of those policies. Furthermore, prevention education programs and related approaches specific to an area or subpopulation must be designed, implemented, and continuously evaluated. There are many reasons that community-based efforts are vital to complement broader policy and programs, including the power that comes from local people having a sense of ownership of and therefore commitment to the intervention that is launched.

Both levels of intervention, national/provincial/state and regional/local, require effective leadership. There are those at the highest level who need to manage "diversion channels" and thereby reduce the level of a flood, and there are those leaders who need to come alongside local animators and community members and inspire, guide, and coordinate efforts to "fill sandbags" and situate them strategically to minimize flood damage.

This book is primarily about leaders fulfilling the latter, more localized role in chronic disease prevention.

In most of the discussion to follow, these regional/local leaders will be referred to as community-based prevention educators (CPEs). Different terms for the role have been used in different jurisdictions and contexts, such as *cancer control specialist, chronic disease prevention educator, chronic disease prevention strategy educator, health promotion officer,* and *community-based chronic disease educator.*

Specifically, the prevention, treatment, and monitoring program supported by the ongoing operating budget of the taxpayer-supported cancer agency in British Columbia – another province situated, like Manitoba, in the western part of Canada – uses the term *Prevention Educational Leader* to refer to its staff. The program in British Columbia was the original inspiration for the project that led to this book.

Purpose of the Book

Given the preceding context, the two purposes of this book are:

- To understand the rationale for looking more closely at community-based prevention educators, and the practice, complexities, and potential benefits of the role as it operates in programs around the world
- To abstract important elements or principles of a CPE program that will inspire and inform policy-makers and planners who might be considering such a strategy in their organization or jurisdiction

With this purpose in view, it is appropriate to begin unpacking the core theme of the book, namely, the community-based prevention educator.

CPE: A First Look

Before reviewing cancer, chronic disease, and other CPE-related framing contexts in more detail in the next chapter, the balance of this chapter will outline the basic role description of a CPE.

Prologue: A Real Life Example of a CPE in Action

Mark (names have been changed) recently made a decision that he had wanted to make for a long time. He chose to try to take control of his health, in particular to live a more active and healthy lifestyle. The initial decision was easy, but putting it into action and sticking with it took more effort. Fortunately, his community had the support of Susan, who indirectly became Mark's ally. Through using tools such as an Environmental Scan and Needs Assessment as well as being well networked and involved in local committees, Susan helped the community where Mark lived in a variety of ways. For instance, she had identified the necessity of providing safe walking and running trails with appropriate signage, as well as drawing attention to opportunities for outside sponsorship. The resulting collaborative initiative that grew out of these actions came to be called "Healthy Actions 4 Life." It included members from the local health authority, school district, parks and recreation, tourism, Chamber of Commerce, sporting groups, Rotary Club, and other entities. The group worked to create a Community Action Plan, which soon evolved to include Susan taking on an active role in promoting exercise in schools and after-school, workplace wellness programs, community activity and healthy eating campaigns, point of decision signage, policy development, and large community-based celebration events to showcase activities, raise awareness about healthy lifestyle choices, and recognize community champions.

The sight of many other people walking, cycling, running, and choosing wholesome foods is a stimulus for those sitting on the fence about getting active and making healthy choices; it all contributes to building a healthier community, which in turn reinforces and perpetuates the healthy activities and, most importantly, teaches new generations to adopt such a lifestyle. It normalizes healthy behaviours. Because of this gradual shift, Mark was helped by a community-wide effort to make his healthy choices the easy choice; as a consequence, he is well on his way to achieving his goals. This is a remarkable phenomenon, especially when one considers that Mark and Susan have never actually met or spoken. Susan is a community-based prevention educator, a category of health care worker charged with the complicated task of encouraging and facilitating preventive health care across a whole community. She understands how difficult it is to change ingrained behaviours, but she is also aware of the health and economic consequences if behaviour changes are not made. Increasing rates of chronic disease can be largely attributed to rising obesity rates, fewer people being physically active or eating well, and the substantial proportion of the population that still smokes.

The prevention of chronic diseases is critical to reducing health care costs. Reflective of this, Susan is attacking the problem from the ground up – working to catalyse pre-existing community structures, including not-for-profit organizations and service groups, and to establish new ones in order to create an environment that encourages and facilitates individuals like Mark to make the changes that are required to prevent disease and to have a better quality of life. Susan lives in the same community as Mark, and understands the unique nuances of the community and how to go about getting things done – things like the creation of safe jogging trails, encouraging residents to walk for short errands, and enabling other changes so that the healthy choice becomes the easy choice. This process empowers individuals to take a proactive approach to their health rather than a reactive one that only deals with illness after it has occurred. Through partnerships with local, regional, provincial, and national organizations, Susan is facilitating community-wide changes, while helping to provide educational and other opportunities aimed at supporting motivated individuals and the population at large, now and well into the future.

The scenario above, inspired by a true event, offers a glimpse of what a prevention educational leader program looks like as it exists in British Columbia, Canada, as well as previewing similar efforts in other parts of the world. As implied in the description, the prevention focus of the program is cancer and other chronic diseases, many of which share similar risk factors, including tobacco use, obesity, poor diet, and a lack of exercise. These factors represent a key focus for a CPE-type program.

Definition of a CPE

To begin understanding the CPE role in more general terms, the following definition may be abstracted from sources describing CPEs as they are constituted in British Columbia, the program that prompted this book:

> A CPE is a professional leader coordinating community-based efforts to reduce the common risk factors and/or progression of cancer and other chronic diseases in a defined population.

This definition firmly locates CPEs at the public or community health end of the health care spectrum, in contrast to approaches related to primary and other types of care delivered by clinicians. However, the prevention strategies encompassed by public health represent a very broad arena involving different kinds of leadership. In this light, it is important to recognize that there are important dimensions that characterize CPEs and distinguish them from other types of prevention workers.

Characteristics of the CPE Program

First, even if hired on a part-time basis, a CPE is clearly a *professional*, notably because the role entails a broad scope of work that requires a demanding skill set involving leading and/or facilitating the work of others. Of course, there is also the basic practical fact that a CPE is paid rather than acting as a volunteer.

The next dimension starts with the idea of *community*, a word that can mean so many things that it immediately calls for some definition. CPEs are in fact community-focused in a variety of ways. They are community-based; there is a defined boundary around the *population* to which they are assigned and whose health they are trying to influence for the better. The boundary is usually geographical – in other words, the CPEs work in a particular region, but it may also entail a combination of geographical and ethnocultural factors (e.g., all people of Chinese ethnicity in an area). The aspect that links these two types of groupings is that everyone in the community is included: all ages, both sexes, all socioeconomic levels, etc. CPEs are also community-focused in the sense that the strategies they promote are generally meant to have an impact on the whole community rather than on individuals or a small subset of the population. There can be exceptions, where a specific group (e.g., youth, immigrants, the poor) may be the focus of a particular initiative, but, ultimately all members of a community are included in the defined population target of the CPE. As noted earlier, this characteristic scope means that CPEs may be distinguished from clinical staff working with clients in the one-to-one, face-to-face manner that is customary in a primary care setting.

The word "community" occurs in the third dimension of the role as well, in terms of the main strategic framework for the CPE. This may be summed up as community engagement and capacity building. Consistent with the goal of improving the health of the whole population in a region, CPEs typically work towards mobilizing the community from the ground up. It is clear that their education function entails far more than passive teaching and learning. The aim is to have as many people in a community, both grassroots members and their representatives, actively engaged in the process of improving population health, and to ensure that the community becomes a partner in the process of evolving and sustaining the opportunities for healthy lifestyle choices over time. This approach may be contrasted with a pure "program delivery" model, where a certain plan created in an office far away is imported into (and to some extent imposed on) the target region. In reality, there will likely be a degree of program "marketing" and management included in CPE work, but always in a nuanced fashion that pays close attention to all the local contexts and leaders. Likewise, time spent cooperating with other coordinators – to influence broader policies or plans or to create general materials or programs – is always balanced with the main goal of targeting health improvement in a particular area of the province or in a specific demographic subset.

Finally, CPEs act as *generalists* in their education/promotion function and other prevention leadership. One example of an inclusive strategy is the fact that both primary prevention (reducing risk factors) and secondary prevention (screening for disease precursors) are appropriate areas of focus for a CPE. Further, when primary prevention is the target, then all of the five key preventable cancer risk factors are on the agenda, including tobacco use; physical inactivity; excess calories leading to obesity; the absence of, for instance, vegetables and fruits in the diet; and overexposure to ultraviolet radiation. Education concerning each risk factor is not provided in isolation, which enables a more powerful message to be conveyed and creates an opportunity for cross-promotion based on the fact that the large majority of preventable risk factors for cancer (all except overexposure to ultraviolet radiation) are also linked with other chronic diseases – with the underlying message for the public being that reducing the risk for cancer also leads to a reduction in the risk of other chronic diseases.

In sum, while CPEs may bring some unique background and specific expertise to their assignment, the broader perspective must always be in front of them. However, despite the generalist nature of the position, there are still some limits to the assigned task. For instance, a useful distinction may be drawn between behavioural and biological risk factors. The first set includes smoking, inactivity, unhealthy diet, and (in the case of cancer) excessive ultraviolet radiation exposure, while the latter includes high cholesterol, hypertension, and severe obesity. It is interesting to note that the biological risk conditions are sometimes considered diseases in their own right. Generally, the behavioural or lifestyle matters are the main purview of the CPE. Monitoring cholesterol levels and hypertension across a population may be part of the evaluation of interventions; however, a clinical/medical approach to chronic conditions, while useful, is usually *not* part of the strategies being promoted by CPEs as it goes beyond their area of expertise.

The preceding four dimensions of the CPE role will be revisited in a latter part of the book, specifically in the context of identifying case studies that may be considered comparable to a CPE-type program.

Plan of the Book

Part A: Purpose and Context

Having already introduced the purpose of the book and begun to characterize the basic picture of a community-based prevention educator, it will be useful to further underline the potential significance of the

CPE model. Part A provides additional context by unpacking core elements of cancer and chronic diseases and their prevention, combined with further perspectives on being a community-based educator focusing on those themes. Next, the "touchstone" for the book, the CPE-type program operating in British Columbia, Canada, will be introduced in some detail.

Part B: Other Models of Community-Based Prevention Educators

In order to provide the grid by which to choose comparable programs that can serve as useful case studies, Part B begins by further characterizing what a prevention educator is – and is not. In the end, five jurisdictions were identified as having one or more programs similar to that of the CPEs in British Columbia: Finland, Northern Ireland, Kentucky, North Carolina, and Manitoba. A similar pattern was followed for each case study, first describing the background and operation of the program, then making comparisons with the original exemplar in British Columbia, and finally abstracting insights applicable to any CPE-type strategy.

Part C: A Strategic Pattern for Prevention Educators

The last part of the book begins with a précis of the insights gleaned from an assessment of the CPE program in British Columbia and from the analyses in the various case studies. It is important to recall that the picture of a prevention educator was first established *inductively* from the program in British Columbia, with strategic insights for implementing or improving such a program then elaborated from models in other jurisdictions. In other words, the picture was developed from a "real world" context rather than abstractly from theory.

Even though the strategic pattern identified did not depend on deductive reasoning based on theory, there are profitable complementary insights that can be learned from the academic literature. The most critical areas of additional research related to one element that was present in most programs, namely, the application of a *conceptual framework* or *theory of practice*, plus one element that was an identified gap in most cases, that is, a robust commitment to *evaluation*. After two chapters offering background on these specific areas, the concluding chapter pulls together the main themes of the book, and ends by reflecting on the investment that is required to make population-level progress on reducing the burden of cancer and chronic diseases.

Information Sources for the Project

Each part of the book has its own profile in terms of sources. For Part A, the background on cancer, chronic diseases, community, and education is drawn from the scientific literature. Here the convention is introduced that is followed throughout the book, namely, to offer a brief reading list of sources and other pertinent material for the reader who wants to delve deeper. The aim is to avoid an overly academic feel by avoiding copious footnotes.

The major chapter on the CPEs in British Columbia was developed from historical program materials on file at the B.C. Cancer Agency, augmented by formal publications. Another very productive source involved feedback from existing CPEs made available through responses to surveys, discussion at a semi-annual gathering of CPEs, and selected one-to-one interviews. Appendix I identifies the respondents who contributed in this way.

The prevention educator case studies in Part B were initially developed from the information, sometimes quite extensive, available at official sites or in the scientific literature. The various interviews conducted with leaders from the various international programs were a fruitful source of information and insight. Again, Appendix I provides a list of the informants consulted.

Finally, most of the material in Part C is intentionally drawn from the broader literature. The aim is to offer an illuminating perspective on the particularities discovered in the case studies. All of the lines of evidence are intended to come together in a pattern that planners of a CPE-type program can follow in order to effectively address cancer and chronic diseases in their particular setting.

Sources and Further Reading

H. Krueger & Associates Inc. *Making the Case for Primary Prevention: An Economic Analysis of Risk Factors in Manitoba*. 2010. Available at http://krueger.ca/index.asp?Page=Projects (accessed 10 January 2010).

Milken Institute. *An Unhealthy America: The Economic Burden of Chronic Disease*. 2007. Available at http://www.milkeninstitute.org/publications/ (accessed 15 February 2010).

National Center for Chronic Disease Prevention and Health Promotion. *The Power of Prevention*. 2009. Available at http://www.cdc.gov/chronicdisease/overview/pop.htm (accessed 8 February 2010).

Nolte E, McKee C. *Measuring the Health of Nations: Updating an Earlier Analysis.* 2008. Available at http://www.commonwealthfund.org/ (accessed 23 January 2010).

Ormond BA, Spillman BC, Waidmann TA, et al. Potential national and state medical care savings from primary disease prevention. Am J Public Health. 2011;101(1):157–64. http://dx.doi.org/10.2105/AJPH.2009.182287. Medline:21088270

Quam L, Smith R, Yach D. Rising to the global challenge of the chronic disease epidemic. Lancet. 2006;368(9543):1221–3. http://dx.doi.org/10.1016/S0140-6736(06)69422-1. Medline:17027712

Thomas A, Rees M. Identifying and preventing chronic disease in an ageing world. Maturitas. 2010;65(2):85–6. http://dx.doi.org/10.1016/j.maturitas.2009.12.016. Medline:20036787

Trust for Health. *Prevention for a Healthier America: Investments in Disease Prevention Yield Significant Savings, Strong Communities.* 2008. Available at http://healthyamericans.org (accessed 15 February 2010).

2 Cancer, Chronic Disease, and the Relevance of CPEs

As was introduced in the first chapter, addressing the burden of cancer and other chronic diseases is an urgent matter. For many countries, thousands of lives, millions of disability-adjusted life years, and billions of dollars are at stake.

Fortunately, there are some strategic "pluses" related to chronic disease that may be exploited by prevention efforts. One "advantage" for prevention educators is that many of the chronic diseases share important risk factors; notably, these include tobacco use, obesity, poor diet, and a lack of exercise. More than half of cancer deaths, for instance, can be prevented by modifying these risk factors.

Chronic diseases are also generally marked by slow progression or frequent recurrence, and therefore tend to affect the afflicted individual over a longer period of time. From a biological perspective, a chronic disease characteristically persists beyond the normal period wherein damaged tissue might naturally heal. From the medical perspective, this type of disease can be controlled or managed but usually not cured (otherwise it would not be *chronic*). The chronic category is usually contrasted with acute diseases, which are characterized by rapid onset and/or a short duration before either a cure or death is realized. Compared to acute conditions, the further "advantage" of a chronic disease is the fact that its slower development allows more opportunity to interrupt the exposure to or consequences of a risk factor.

Cancer offers a nuanced example of these principles. Tumour formation usually entails a slow process involving the accumulation of damage to many genes; the damage may be promoted by certain risk factors (sometimes unique to cancer) and exploited by other risk factors that are often common to chronic disease. Once diagnosed, a case of cancer

can sometimes be quickly cured by surgical excision or other thera-
peutic intervention. Other cases progress quickly to death. Still other
cancers become truly chronic, controlled by treatment but not cured.
Survival in the latter instance can last for decades, with eventual death
sometimes occurring from another cause altogether. In sum, cancer can
manifest as either an acute or a chronic disease. Cancer can be legitimately included in a discussion of chronic disease because an increasing proportion of previously unsalvageable cancer patients are being
diagnosed earlier and responding to new therapies – a phenomenon
made possible by the generally slow causal process driven by common
chronic disease risk factors.

It is useful to continue establishing the context for this book by addressing the general significance of the topic. Four key concepts are
suggested in the book's title:

- Cancer (prevention)
- Chronic disease (prevention)
- Community
- Education

These terms provide a helpful guide to the motivations and main themes
addressed in the book. For this reason, each concept will be briefly examined to offer further background. The discussion to follow essentially
answers the question: *Why be motivated to recruit and deploy CPEs?*

Cancer, the focus of the British Columbia Cancer Agency prevention
program that inspired this project, provides a natural starting point,
to be followed with an examination of chronic disease as a whole. It
has already been made very clear that chronic diseases represent major
challenges facing higher income countries and, increasingly, the lower
and middle income world. The reality of the burden will be explored
further in two major sections to follow. This will lead to a reflection on
complex themes already introduced, namely, how being community-
based interacts with a specific educational role that will enable a population to make progress on the burden of cancer and other chronic
disease.

Cancer: A Major Prevention Opportunity

Even though there are signs of progress, the battle against cancer is certainly not over. Globally, there were some 12 million people diagnosed

with cancer in 2008, the latest year that such information was compiled and reported. This is a substantial number by any standard, but the level of personal fear related to cancer is greater than the bare statistics indicate. The progress of malignancies can be insidious, treatments are often debilitating, and recurrence is common. Although developments in life-extending therapies have been remarkable, survival rates remain low for many types of cancer. Even in a well-resourced country such as Canada, less than two-thirds of all people who experience cancer are alive after 5 years. There are certain cancers in that country that have alarmingly low 5-year survival rates, including stomach (23%), liver (18%), lung (15%), and esophagus (14%). Taking all types of the disease together, over 10% of mortality in the world is attributable to cancer. The figure is even higher in the high-income world, where, for instance, acute infection as a cause of death is much lower.

Cancer has been a traditional focus of medical care in high-income countries, with certain cancers dominating the agenda. In fact, at least 1 in 10 deaths in these jurisdictions are due to just four types of cancer: lung, colorectal, breast, and stomach. But concerns about cancer are no longer limited to Western, industrialized countries; indeed, the majority of the global cancer burden is now found in low- and medium-income countries. This means that there are few people in the world who are not touched directly or indirectly by cancer. A summary taken from the *World Cancer Report* of 2008 helps to clarify the issues facing the whole world:

> Hardly any family has not been hit by cancer, and when cancer hits it can hit hard. The burden on society caused by cancer is immense not only in terms of the human suffering of patients and their relatives and friends, but the cost of cancer in economic terms. The strain cancer produces on health professionals and health systems is substantial and growing rapidly.

In addition to direct health care costs, cancer is a very common cause of impoverishment as families lose a bread winner and/or try to pay for out-of-pocket expenses related to treatments that are too often unsuccessful.

It is estimated that the number of new cancer cases doubled in the last three decades of the twentieth century, will double again in the period between 2000 and 2020, and will nearly triple by 2030. The growing burden of cancer is driven mostly by demographic forces, specifically the expansion and ageing of populations. In a few cases, changes in underlying risk factors are involved. For instance, although oral cancers should be declining in areas where tobacco use is decreasing, the role of another causal factor, *human papillomavirus* infection, is helping to keep the number of new cases elevated.

The picture provided here of the current and future burden of cancer should be enough to inspire the establishment of a program of community-based prevention educators (CPEs). But the real reason to pursue such a strategy is even more compelling: quite simply, based on present knowledge, a large percentage of cancer is actually *preventable*. According to the leading international experts, by removing modifiable risk factors such as smoking, unhealthy diet, and physical inactivity, at least 50% of cancer cases could be eliminated. And this is not merely a theoretical claim. When population-wide risk factor changes have been achieved within a jurisdiction, cancer rates have indeed declined. One of the most dramatic examples of this pattern has been seen with tobacco smoking and lung cancer in countries such as Canada (as demonstrated in Figure 2.1, focusing on males).

It is important to note that there was a 20-year lag time before an effect on lung cancer rates was observed; this reflects the latency period following carcinogen exposure and prior to the emergence of disease. Such patterns underline both the urgency and challenge of cancer prevention efforts. On one hand, it is important to stem the tide as soon as possible because positive impacts may be a generation or more away. On the other, it may be difficult to garner the necessary level of political attention and support when several election cycles must elapse before full benefits are made manifest. At a societal level, this is one explanation for the generally slow and, to be generous, often modest policy responses in the arena of cancer prevention. Another factor is the "knowledge translation" gap. Information about the preventability of cancer is not always presented clearly and forcefully to policymakers – and neither is the evidence for the effectiveness of specific risk factor interventions. Furthermore, there often are delays in implementing effective interventions in the real world.

In short, there is a gap between the known science and its application. If this is true for health care planners, then it is worse for ordinary people. A degree of fatalism persists about the unavoidability of tumours, especially when there is a family history of cancer. There is also sometimes a surprising lack of awareness of modifiable risk factors. For example, over a quarter of respondents in a recent Health Information

Figure 2.1. Prevalence of Daily Smokers and Age-Standardized Lung Cancer Incidents: Males, Canada.

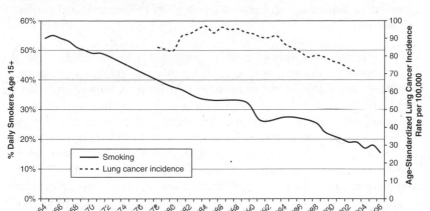

National Trends Survey in the United States agreed that "there's not much people can do to lower their chances of getting cancer."

The truth lies in the opposite direction. Because up to half of all cancer cases can be prevented by implementing what is known today about modifying risk factors, it is disconcerting that over 70% of respondents in the same survey perceived that "there are so many recommendations about preventing cancer, it's hard to know which ones to follow." Given this context, there clearly is a large window of opportunity for CPEs to be active in health education and health promotion, offering solid evidence-based information to the general public and policymakers alike.

As already suggested, the cancer crisis is a global reality. Prevention is especially important in low- and medium-resource countries, where cancer treatment facilities are not universally available. As noted once again in the 2008 *World Cancer Report*,

> A major issue for many countries, even among high-resource countries, will be how to find sufficient funds to treat all cancer patients effectively and provide palliative, supportive and terminal care for the large numbers of patients, and their relatives, who will be diagnosed in the coming years.... Translational research in its broadest sense is of paramount ·

importance to cancer control, covering the spectrum from translating cut-
ting-edge scientific discovery into new approaches to cancer treatment to
translating knowledge of cancer risk factors into changes in population
behaviour.

The need for such learning transfer from science to the field is vital in
wealthy and developing countries alike. Among the many roles that
they may play, CPEs are in an excellent position to act as "knowledge
translation specialists" in the regions where they are based.

It is important to acknowledge that sharing information about risk
factors for cancer (and other chronic diseases) is not enough to change
behaviours. A sample of Canadians in British Columbia surveyed by
Environics Research Group in 2008 generated the following stark picture: Two-thirds of the respondents said they were too busy to exercise,
and just over half said they were too busy to prepare healthier food.
This further underlines the necessity and challenge of intensifying action at many levels of society, including the local community.

Chronic Disease: A Growing Burden Driven by Common Risk Factors

Cancer is but one of several chronic diseases of concern in both the
higher-income and lower- and middle-income world. An elevated
level of concern is certainly warranted. For example, data from 2005
show that 7 of the 10 leading causes of death in the United States were
chronic diseases; in addition to cancer, they included cardiovascular
disease, stroke, chronic lower respiratory diseases, diabetes, and kidney disease, all of which are modifiable to some extent. Chronic diseases also account for significant morbidity, from extended pain and
suffering to various levels of disability, with each condition leading to
its own set of limitations on the activities of daily living.

Cardiovascular disease (CVD) continues to dominate among the
causes of mortality. For example, CVD, which includes heart attacks
(also known as acute myocardial infarctions) and stroke, is one of the
leading global causes of death. In Canada, it is the underlying cause of
one out of every three deaths.

Once considered "diseases of prosperity" because of their strong link
to unhealthy diet and physical inactivity, CVD and other chronic diseases
are now common in low- and middle-income countries as well. In fact,
80% of global deaths due to chronic non-communicable diseases occur in

these settings. Thus, there is a good argument to see the work of prevention extended beyond the high-income world. This enhancement of the agenda is made easier because there is a substantial overlap between the risk factors for cancer and those associated with other chronic diseases, a theme that will be explored further in the next subsection.

Common Risk Factors

A collateral benefit of prevention efforts directed at cancer or one of the major chronic diseases is the potential reduction of certain other chronic diseases. This phenomenon directly relates to the *common* modifiable risk factors shared by cancer and chronic diseases. The key causal factors related to the various diseases include tobacco use and physical inactivity, as well as different aspects of an unhealthy diet – with excess alcohol consumption representing a special instance of dietary intake. The main risk factor information in the current literature is summarized in Table 2.1.

It is important to note that this inventory will undoubtedly be expanded as research continues. One emerging area involves the link between infection and many cancers, as well as the growing evidence that some cases of other chronic diseases may be linked to infection-based inflammatory processes.

Synergistic Efforts

Acknowledging the modifiable risk factors with overlapping associations to two or more diseases is akin to recognizing the synergistic potential of prevention, that is, a key opportunity for enhanced education and engagement outcomes. In short, educators specializing in cancer prevention will make an impact on other chronic diseases; while the same may be said of prevention specialists for CVD and other chronic disease, the emotionally charged topic of cancer occupies a unique position in the public mind. Due to the prevalence of cancer and the severity of the typical treatment process, many people will be particularly inclined to take note of information regarding how to prevent it. At such times, CPEs can mention the other chronic diseases that can also be prevented through the same lifestyle choices that relate to the modifiable risk factors for cancer prevention. Having similar messaging originating from various perspectives and organizations is a powerful tool for educating and encouraging people to make healthy lifestyle choices.

Table 2.1 Risk Factor Overlap for Various Diseases

Disease	Smoking	Physical Inactivity	Alcohol	Dietary			
				Low Fruit + Vegetable Intake	High Saturated Fat Intake	High Salt Intake	Excess Caloric Intake
Cancer	•	•	•	•		•	•
Cardiovascular Disease	•	•		•	•	•	•
Alzheimer's Disease	•	•		•	•	•	
Chronic Kidney Disease	•	•				•	•
Stroke	•	•			•	•	•
Diabetes (Type II)	•	•			•		•

The phenomenon of common risk factors enhances the public health benefit of a CPE and creates a foundation for natural alliances with health organizations focusing on other chronic diseases. A perfect example of this would be a partnership between societies with a focus on heart, lungs, or cancer and dietician/diabetes associations and interest groups, with all of the above further linked to associations of municipalities, amateur sports groups, and so on. Such a linkage has occurred in British Columbia under the name of the B.C. Healthy Living Alliance. There are many examples of such alliances or coalitions around the world. One of the achievements of such a partnership involved a planning exercise for the province that ultimately was chronicled in a 2007 University of Toronto Press book, *The Health Impact of Smoking and Obesity and What to Do about It.*

Community: A Platform for Success

Beyond the disease burden that provides a strong mandate for the work of CPEs and similar leaders, the inherent community foundation of that work is also an important part of the picture. "Community" is a difficult word to define. Reviewing the actual practice of the CPEs in British Columbia helps to navigate through the various meanings of the term. Their role will be described further in the next chapter of the book, but the pertinent points can be briefly raised here to begin to illustrate just how important prevention educators can be in the cause of reducing chronic disease.

The meaning of community that applies in the case of CPEs is first of all geographical. The CPEs are a regionalized force in British Columbia – a province in the west of Canada consisting of 4.5 million people. The population enjoys a single-payer approach to physician compensation and a hospital system that is government controlled. The CPEs are assigned to different parts of the province and in fact are usually hired from the target area. The regions vary in physical size, but the geographical organizing principle remains the same. In the cases where CPEs are asked to specialize within a cultural group, they are located where established clusters of recent immigrants reside and become content specialists for the rest of the CPE group.

There is a second way to understand community that also applies to the work of CPEs. It stresses the relationship or "commonality" aspects of community. In short, CPEs not only operate *within* a community, but precisely by means of *building* community. This concept is closely allied with the idea of coordination, which will be addressed further in the next section. Prevention educators are community organizers; this involves fostering relationships and common understanding – specifically a sense of teamwork and a deeper insight with respect to prevention strategy for a region. The people involved with this secondary expression of community theoretically coincides with all the residents of a region, but in practical terms the application is narrower, referring to those who are actively concerned about and engaged in a common, population-wide prevention plan for the sake of the broader community. In summary, CPEs are engaged in building a community (of mobilized people) for the sake of the community (of all citizens).

The idea of a geographical community reinforces a CPE-type approach by exploiting the inherent wisdom in a "divide-and-conquer" prevention strategy, covering the needs of a province or state in a regionalized way. The advantages are manifold. First, it is simply easier to conceptualize (and, ideally, to measure) a smaller, more compact group of people as the target of health improvement. Further, it is easier to travel around and meet with local leaders, to identify local needs, and to tailor potential solutions in the context of local issues and human resources. Finally, the existing social connections are more extensive, and informal communication channels are better established, allowing for advertising and training budgets to be stretched while still producing useful results.

Education as Coordination: An Effective Approach

A hallmark of the CPE role is suggested by its very title, namely, being an educator. This core involves education through both classic teaching/training platforms (i.e., coordinating and delivering information) and broader expressions of organizational coordination. There are several recognized advantages of community-based organizing that aims at coordinating multiple lines of information, multiple players, and multiple agendas. This approach has been found to:

• Acknowledge the complex pattern of players that contribute to
  population health (as illustrated in Figure 2.2, adapted from a 2009
  paper in the journal *Global Health Promotion*)
• Mobilize the energies of different formal and informal leaders and
  networks in order to accomplish a large task

- Reflect the fact that community problems are complex and have multifaceted causes
- Facilitate the multiple interventions that are required to affect individual behaviours and the socioeconomic environment within which personal decisions are made, recognizing that there is no option but to pursue an integrated approach to the challenge being faced
- Strengthen the social networks of community members and leaders that come together to effect change and improve health, in this way inspiring broader cohesiveness that helps to create a climate for ideas to spread, be reinforced, and cause "viral" change
- Sustain prevention programs because they are designed or at least adapted locally
- Create interventions that can be very cost-effective; one needs only to compare the impact of an activity campaign with a 1% success rate delivered to a community of 50,000 with the costs and results for a set of exercise classes involving a total of 500 participants – even if the latter program had 50 times the success rate, the community program would still be twice as successful!

A final consideration is required concerning the twin themes of community and education/coordination. Because of the sponsorship and purpose of the project that led to this book, the emphasis will be on the educator role and the coordination work that it accomplishes within a particular community. The emphasis could have been the other way around, taking "community" as an organizing principle. This would have led to a very different book, and a dilution of the focus on CPEs. In fact, there are several other community-based prevention approaches, including:

- Community-oriented primary care (a variation on the theme of primary health care, and demonstrating overlaps with well-known chronic care model)
- Health-promoting hospitals
- Lay health workers
- Creating a very broad collaboration of local policy-makers from different social arenas, not just health care but also agricultural policy, transportation planning, public education, municipal government, industry, and so on.

Figure 2.2. Societal Influencers of Population Health.

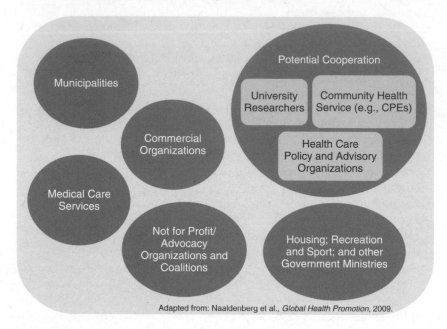

Potential Cooperation

Municipalities

University Researchers

Community Health Service (e.g., CPEs)

Commercial Organizations

Health Care Policy and Advisory Organizations

Medical Care Services

Not for Profit/ Advocacy Organizations and Coalitions

Housing; Recreation and Sport; and other Government Ministries

Adapted from: Naaldenberg et al., *Global Health Promotion*, 2009.

As defined, it is beyond the scope of this book to explore each of these other models of community-based prevention in detail. It must suffice to say that although prevention educators may be in some way connected to each of these models, they demonstrate a unique set of features and benefits.

Summary

This chapter has identified four overlapping rationales for pursuing a closer examination of CPEs. They are as follows:

- The unique burden of cancer and the importance of its prevention; there has been population-level progress on cancer and other chronic diseases, which is certainly encouraging, but much more effort is needed
- The interrelationship between factors that influence cancer risk and other chronic diseases suggests the potential for powerful prevention synergies

- The geographical community and a regionalized effort in community-building is a useful strategy by which to make advances in the prevention battle
- The potentially effective role to be played by those with an educational perspective combined with a coordination approach

The foundation has now been laid to pursue in more detail the manner in which CPEs in the British Columbia context have been motivated and shaped by these rationales, before turning to comparable programs that were identified in different parts of the world.

Sources and Further Reading

Rationale Related to Cancer

American Institute for Cancer Research/World Cancer Research Fund. *Policy and Action for Cancer Prevention.* Available at http://www.preventcanceraicr.org/site/PageServer?pagename=research_science_policy_report (accessed 15 February 2010).

Canadian Cancer Society. *Canadian Cancer Statistics 2011.* Available at http://www.cancer.ca (accessed July 2011).

Environics Research Group. *Cancer Prevention – Attitudes. Awareness and Behaviours – A Survey of Residents of British Columbia.* 2009.

H. Krueger and Associates Inc. *An Overview of Selected Cancers and Modifiable Cancer Risk Factors in Canada.* 2008. Available at http://www.krueger.ca/index.asp?Page=Projects#StatusReport (accessed 23 February 2010).

International Agency for Research on Cancer. *World Cancer Report.* 2008. Available at http://www.iarc.fr/en/publications/pdfs-online/wcr/2008/index.php (accessed 8 February 2010).

Niederdeppe J, Levy AG. Fatalistic beliefs about cancer prevention and three prevention behaviors. Cancer Epidemiol Biomarkers Prev. 2007;16(5):998–1003. http://dx.doi.org/10.1158/1055-9965.EPI-06-0608. Medline:17507628

Rabin BA, Glasgow RE, Kerner JF, et al. Dissemination and implementation research on community-based cancer prevention: a systematic review. Am J Prev Med. 2010;38(4):443–56. http://dx.doi.org/10.1016/j.amepre.2009.12.035. Medline:20307814

Senn HJ, Kerr D. Chronic non-communicable diseases, the European Chronic Disease Alliance – and cancer. Ann Oncol. 2011;22(2):248–9. http://dx.doi.org/10.1093/annonc/mdq753. Medline:21278221

Rationale Related to Chronic Disease and Common Risk Factors

Heart and Stroke Foundation of Canada. *The Growing Burden of Heart Disease and Stroke 2003*. Available at http://www.cvdinfobase.ca/cvdbook/CVD_En03.pdf (accessed 15 February 2010).

International Diabetes Federation, World Heart Federation, International Union Against Cancer. *Time to Act: The Global Emergency of Non-Communicable Diseases.* 2009.

Izzotti A, Durando P, Ansaldi F, et al. Interaction between Helicobacter pylori, diet, and genetic polymorphisms as related to non-cancer diseases. Mutat Res. 2009;667(1-2):142–57. http://dx.doi.org/10.1016/j.mrfmmm.2009.02.002. Medline:19563929

Kahn R, Robertson RM, Smith R, et al. The impact of prevention on reducing the burden of cardiovascular disease. Diabetes Care. 2008;31(8):1686–96. http://dx.doi.org/10.2337/dc08-9022. Medline:18663233

Krueger H, Stuart G, Gallagher R, et al. *HPV and Other Infectious Agents in Cancer: Opportunities for Prevention and Public Health.* New York: Oxford University Press; 2010.

Krueger H, Williams D, Kaminsky B, et al. *The Health Impact of Smoking and Obesity and What to Do about It.* Toronto: University of Toronto Press; 2007.

Lee DS, Chiu M, Manuel DG, et al., and the Canadian Cardiovascular Outcomes Research Team. Trends in risk factors for cardiovascular disease in Canada: temporal, socio-demographic and geographic factors. CMAJ. 2009;181(3-4):E55–66. http://dx.doi.org/10.1503/cmaj.081629. Medline:19620271

Mahmoudi M, Curzen N, Gallagher PJ. Atherogenesis: the role of inflammation and infection. Histopathology. 2007;50(5):535–46. http://dx.doi.org/10.1111/j.1365-2559.2006.02503.x. Medline:17394488

Manuel DG, Leung M, Nguyen K, et al., and the Canadian Cardiovascular Outcomes Research Team. Burden of cardiovascular disease in Canada. Can J Cardiol. 2003;19(9):997–1004. Medline:12915926

Nusselder WJ, Franco OH, Peeters A, et al. Living healthier for longer: comparative effects of three heart-healthy behaviors on life expectancy with and without cardiovascular disease. BMC Public Health. 2009;9(1):487. http://dx.doi.org/10.1186/1471-2458-9-487. Medline:20034381

Ramsey F, Ussery-Hall A, Garcia D, et al. Prevalence of selected risk behaviors and chronic disease – Behavioral Risk Factor Surveillance System (BRFSS), 39 steps communities, Centers for Disease Control and Prevention (CDC). MMWR Surveill Summ. 2008;57(11):1–20.

van Dieren S, Beulens JW, van der Schouw YT, et al. The global burden of diabetes and its complications: an emerging pandemic. Eur J Cardio-vasc Prev Rehabil. 2010;17(Suppl 1):S3–8. http://dx.doi.org/10.1097/01. hjr.0000368191.86614.5a. Medline:20489418

Rationale Related to Community and Educational Leadership/Coordination

Hanusaik N, O'Loughlin JL, Kishchuk N, et al. Organizational capacity for chronic disease prevention: a survey of Canadian public health organiza-tions. Eur J Public Health. 2010;20(2):195–201. http://dx.doi.org/10.1093/eurpub/ckp140. Medline:19843599

Kegler MC, Rigler J, Honeycutt S. The role of community context in plan-ning and implementing community-based health promotion projects. Eval Program Plann. 2011;34(3):246–53. http://dx.doi.org/10.1016/j.evalprog-plan.2011.03.004. Medline:21555048

Koelen MA, Vaandrager L, Wagemakers A. What is needed for coordinated action for health? Fam Pract. 2008;25(Suppl 1):i25–31. http://dx.doi. org/10.1093/fampra/cmn073. Medline:18936114

Minkler M, Wallerstein N. Improving health through community organization and community building. In: M Minkler, editor. Community Organizing and Community Building for Health. 2nd ed. New Brunswick, New Jersey: Rutgers University Press; 2004.

Naaldenberg J, Vaandrager L, Koelen M, et al. Elaborating on systems think-ing in health promotion practice. Glob Health Promot. 2009;16(1):39–47. http://dx.doi.org/10.1177/1757975908100749. Medline:19276332

Neuhauser L, Sparks L, Villagran MM, et al. The power of community-based health communication interventions to promote cancer prevention and con-trol for at-risk populations. Patient Educ Couns. 2008;71(3):315–8. http:// dx.doi.org/10.1016/j.pec.2008.03.015. Medline:18406096

Nissinen A, Berrios X, Puska P. Community-based noncommunicable disease interventions: lessons from developed countries for developing ones. Bull World Health Organ. 2001;79(10):963–70. Medline:11693979

Wilson MG, Lavis JN, Travers R, et al. Community-based knowledge transfer and exchange: helping community-based organizations link research to ac-tion. Implement Sci. 2010;5(1):33. http://dx.doi.org/10.1186/1748-5908-5-33. Medline:20423486

3 Prevention Educational Leaders in British Columbia

The B.C. Cancer Agency (BCCA) is the public deliverer of cancer-related services in the province of British Columbia; as such, it is similar to other government-run health care providers in the arena of cancer that may be found across Canada. All radiation therapy is delivered by BCCA, and all cancer chemotherapy drugs flow through it, whether delivered by BCCA-operated clinics or by regional health authorities. The BCCA falls under the umbrella of the Provincial Health Services Authority rather than the other regionalized health authorities, reflecting its mandate to provide high-quality services for all citizens in British Columbia who are afflicted with, or at risk for, cancer. All cancer care, including screening programs, is delivered according to peer-developed protocols, ensuring consistency. These efforts, together with other factors at work in the province, have helped to create one of the lowest cancer incidence and mortality rates in North America.

It is fair to say that treatment, research, and secondary prevention (comprised of screening for certain female cancers) dominate the activities of the BCCA; direct spending on chemotherapy drugs and radiation therapy alone represents a third of that agency's budget. In contrast to the long history of comprehensive population-based secondary prevention programs in the province, an active focus on primary prevention of cancer risk factors has been most noticeable in the last decade. Other community groups, mainly disease-based charities, have been involved for a longer period with primary prevention efforts, as have the government tobacco control programs that are now administered by regional health authorities.

In 2007, the BCCA Prevention Programs were awarded the Excellence in Innovation Award by the Canadian College of Health Service Executives in recognition of the approaches and activities that have gone into creating sustainable and measurable benefits for communities. The CPE-type program represents the cornerstone strategy of this successful effort. As noted earlier, the staff persons in this program currently are called Prevention Educational Leaders (PELs).

This chapter of the book has been developed from three main sources:

1 Documents relevant to the program. This includes reports generated for the BCCA, other internal documents, and some published articles.
2 Responses to the survey that was designed specifically for this project; there was a 95% return rate from the PELs. This information was augmented by examining monthly reports submitted by them and additional program materials provided by certain individuals.
3 In-depth interviews with PELs operating in the province.

History of PELs in British Columbia

The origin of the current BCCA CPE-type program may be traced back to 1997, when a donor-funded pilot initiative focusing on the primary prevention of cancer was developed. This pilot project, based in the small city of Vernon, was known as the Waddell Project, a name derived from the benefactor family that provided the initial funding. Representatives from the BCCA Centre for the Southern Interior (CSI), a regional diagnostic and treatment facility, approached the Vernon city council to gain support for a community-based cancer prevention project. Over the following several months word of it spread, resulting in opportunities to speak to and hold discussions with a variety of community organizations. Momentum for the effort grew, and the first part-time Cancer Prevention Coordinator (the title chosen at that time) was hired in April 1999. Even as the project began to be implemented in that initial community, BCCA-CSI representatives were laying the foundation for expansion into the remainder of that catchment area.

Based on a very positive external assessment of the pilot project, ongoing core operating funding was secured to expand the model into the rest of the province, and it is now housed within the Prevention Programs department at BCCA. The most recent development involved adding seven PELs in northern British Columbia so that eventually,

13 years after the initial project planning, there were 20 PELs based in 18 communities covering the various regions of the province (see Figure 3.1). The map shows an unusual geographic distribution of the positions, reflecting the fact that the population of British Columbia is concentrated in the lower coast and in river valleys, with the extensive mountain ranges elsewhere relatively unpopulated.

Vision and Purpose

The motto of prevention programs is "Keeping Healthy People Healthy." Although a simple statement, the task it represents is monumental. There are complexities associated with ensuring that the prevention message is heard and with motivating individuals to take steps to reduce risky behaviours. As well, encouraging community-level changes that support healthy decisions is challenging. Even in the relatively healthy setting represented by British Columbia, it is estimated that at least one in three people will develop cancer over their lifetime; thus, it is likely that no family will remain untouched by the disease. As noted in chapter 2, the good news is that at least 50% of cancers can be prevented through changes in health-related behaviours. The picture is similar for cardiovascular disease and many other common chronic conditions. By engaging with community groups and local stakeholders that share similar goals and objectives, PELs focus on fostering an environment that will support individuals making healthy choices with respect to tobacco use, physical activity, nutrition, and exposure to ultraviolet radiation. Because of the importance of this work, there is an aspirational goal to greatly multiply the current complement of PELs in British Columbia in the years to come.

Organization and Support

Different principles guide the organization of PELs. For example, since one of the sponsored programs related to the PELs is the Healthy Living Schools initiative, it is logical that each PEL is assigned to a specific set of school districts. The main distribution, however, is naturally driven by population centres. The map of the home communities of PELs within British Columbia is shown in Figure 3.1.

Each of five health delivery regions in the province has a lead PEL in the respective major city. The lead PEL is responsible for some supervision of PELs in their region, as well as for interactions with allies in the

Figure 3.1. Regional Distribution of Prevention Educational Leaders (PELs) in British Columbia.

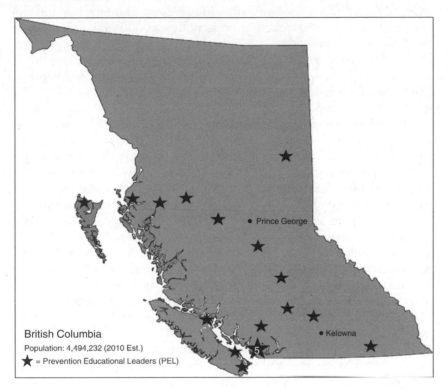

regional health system and other high-level partners. Training of new PELs is both centrally based and managed by the regional lead PEL. In addition, most PELs have a responsibility for shaping one of several province-wide initiatives. These will be reviewed later in the chapter.

Notwithstanding the established structure of responsibility and supervision, there is substantial room for individual initiative. The self-directed nature of the prevention work was characterized by one PEL as follows: "We are not exactly supervised, we are 'advised.' I have really valued the independence this provides me in my work – it is one of the things I love the most about my job." Whether advised or supervised, it is clear that guidance is provided and standards are maintained. The PELs formally report to the Provincial Manager in Vancouver, who is responsible for orienting new PELs and for providing general direction in concert with the Head of Prevention Programs. The latter position is currently held by a physician with a long history of interest in prevention, although the MD qualification is not viewed by the organization as an absolute requirement.

Over the course of the year, the team has two face-to-face meetings, with teleconferences held at least monthly. Outside of these meetings, PELs are also able to contact one another via e-mail and telephone to ask for insight and share expertise. This type of support and input is particularly important for newly recruited PELs; it is in fact an expression of the "teamwork" component of the official PEL role. Many of the PELs noted in their survey responses that being able to learn from more experienced colleagues meant not having to "reinvent the wheel." It also meant avoiding common pitfalls that waste time and energy. One PEL observed the following: "Learning from other PELs is invaluable, I gain confidence as I hear what other PELs are doing, and I also benefit from their creative ideas that have been successful in their towns. Each PEL has their own personal experience, skill set, and regional variances; coming together in person to share these is highly valuable." Maintaining regular communication channels also results in increased awareness of local events about which a PEL may not have heard. This allows the partnerships and knowledge base cultivated by one PEL to be reproduced in another region.

The peer-to-peer encouragement is not the end of the input. Training is offered by internal and invited experts at the face-to-face gatherings. For those PELs that lack an extensive background in health care, the training "curriculum" may be more extensive. One PEL expressed that sentiment in the following way: "Substantial training covering all the content that we're supposed to know, cover, and present to external groups would be most beneficial."

Qualifications

The formal PEL role description involves an extensive inventory of qualifications and requirements (comprising about 40 bullet points). The list was abbreviated to the following highlights in a recent recruiting document:

- 5 to 10 years of experience in community development, health promotion, or capacity-building

- Proactive self-starter with demonstrated skill as a leader, facilitator, innovator, coach, and change agent in a dynamic environment
- University degree(s) in the area of health sciences, social sciences, sciences, public administration, adult education, or related discipline preferred
- Demonstrated excellence in oral and written communication (e.g., public relations, group facilitation, public speaking, writing proposals, articles, and training materials)
- Demonstrated ability to effectively partner and collaborate with other community organizations, to maintain and build partnerships, and to access community resources
- Strong organizational skills, including the ability to assess and manage others effectively, establish clear accountabilities, develop the capabilities of others, and cope effectively with change in complex health care and community systems
- Must value teamwork and collaboration
- Must be comfortable using computer tools (e.g., e-mail, MS Office, databases, and Internet)
- Must have access to a vehicle, be willing and able to travel provincially, and be willing to work outside of normal hours

The PELs currently employed in British Columbia represent a wide variety of backgrounds in terms of life experience, formal education, and work history (see Tables 3.1 and 3.2). Not surprisingly, there is a strong orientation towards helping people, health care, and/or communications. The variety of backgrounds is generally seen to be a strength of the program, as illustrated by the following comment from one PEL: "I think a skill set in conjunction with personal experience is maybe of more value than strict qualifications."

Thus, there is no one credential that is a prerequisite for the PEL role. Although a diploma or degree in health promotion or a related area is not required for the job, the conceptual frameworks associated with health promotion are explicitly embraced by many PELs (see further on this topic in chapter 11). An example of this may be found in the comment from one PEL in northern British Columbia: "The social determinants of health have been part of my consciousness for many years." Similarly, another PEL noted that "community engagement is the most important framework; sustainability of programs in a community can only be accomplished if the individuals living there get involved."

Table 3.1 Key Professional Experience of PELs

Nurse	5
Business Manager	2
School Principal	1
Member of the Legislative Assembly	1
University Lecturer (Sociology)	1
Respiratory Therapist	1
Community Developer in a Health Authority	1
Health and Wellness Consultant	1
Public Health Inspector	1
Career Counsellor	1
Personal Trainer	1
Self-employment Coordinator	1
Media / Television Producer	1
Dietitian	1

Other perspectives and skills also are seen to be valuable, which was aptly summed up in a particular survey response: "You need several skills ... such as excellent written and spoken communication, networking and social skills, engaging the public, public speaking, and confidence are critical to the role of PEL. Others include an ability to work collaboratively, ability to work unsupervised, and delivery of required outcomes, reporting, etc. Understanding and interpreting research also comes into play."

In reality, the PELs have formal training in fields such as nursing, kinesiology, and public health, and typically have years of experience in some form of public administration, volunteer coordination, or project management. The most common professional role in the background of PELs is nursing, represented by about one quarter of the team. However, the key professional experience of PELs extends well beyond health care, including work as a school principal, a broadcaster, and a politician. Importantly, the PEL team also includes cancer survivors.

There is one additional feature; the willingness of the program to hire self-employed contractors if that status is best for the PEL. BCCA accepts that it may be one among a number of clients of the independently

Table 3.2 Highest Degree Achieved by PELs

PhD	
Natural Health Studies	1
Total Masters	1
Nutrition	2
Education	1
Population & Public Health	1
Nursing	1
Sociology	1
Business Administration	1
Total Bachelors	7
Economics	1
Commerce	1
Human Kinetics	1
Nursing	1
Health Sciences (Respiratory Therapy)	1
Total Diploma	5
Nursing	3
Radio/Television Arts	1
Total	4

established business operated by the individual. This acceptance of contractors has several implications in addition to the potential efficiencies and flexibility it offers to the BCCA. First, it means that a PEL can work part-time. Second, it is recognized that a self-starter may not be happy as an employee. Another subtle effect is the difference that exists between a part-time contractor and a full-time government employee; it is arguable that these two types of staff would be accepted in different ways by communities and other community workers. Most critically, being a contractor goes hand-in-hand with working with relative independence. The role description spells out one of the principles of being a contractor, namely, controlling the way work is done and the work methods used. Although limits and expectations do apply, the sense of professional freedom is stated succinctly in recruiting documents, as follows: "Each PEL works independently and ethically with little supervision, adhering to program objectives, processes, and guidelines."

Roles and Responsibilities

Although the activities undertaken by PELs are varied, with each individual bringing their own unique set of skills, interests, and perspectives to the position, there is a core set of responsibilities woven into the fabric of the role. The content and tone of the assignment was captured well by one of the PELs in a survey response, paraphrased as follows:

> The PEL role involves being a *catalyst*, instigator, motivator, collaborator, and (small e) educator. We provide information and tools for people, organizations, and communities to make smarter, healthier choices for themselves, particularly when it comes to cancer prevention. We enlist the help of other groups and organizations to make it possible. And we are to do it in a way that entertains, engages, and inspires.

The official tasks are categorized under four headings, dominated by community action and education (see Figure 3.2). The role description highlights that community action encompasses building and maintaining relationships, as well as fundraising, as necessary to implement and enhance prevention initiatives. Community or public education includes media relations, presentations to public groups, development and/or customization of tools and educational articles, and facilitation of training for health care practitioners. The major role division for PELs appears to reflect the classic distinction drawn between health promotion and health education (see chapter 11 for more on this topic).

For added granularity, two months of status reports chronicling community-based activities were analysed to gain a more detailed perspective on the foci and "platforms" of PEL efforts. The status reports were broken down into two categories:

- **Activity focus:** Classifying each reported activity as either primary prevention or screening. A mixed activity was coded as primary prevention for the sake of the present analysis.
- **Activity platform:** A second classification grouped different program types or settings under two headings – *Core Initiatives* (i.e.,

Figure 3.2. PEL Role Categories by Time Involvement/Emphasis.

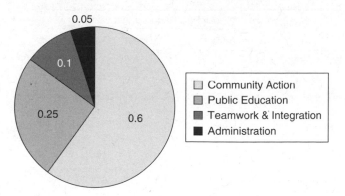

centrally developed programs) and *Other PEL Initiatives* (i.e., activities specific to a region). The details of the various programs are discussed later in this chapter.

Table 3.3 summarizes the results gleaned from the monthly reports, indicative of the proportion of all reported activities that were spent on the specified area. Because of the limited information and time frame, this is admittedly a very rough assessment; there is no attempt to compare the time spent on each area. For example, a PEL spending 4 hours at a health and wellness fair would carry the same weight as a PEL spending 1 hour at a city council meeting.

As might be expected, prevention dominates the picture, reflecting about 90% of the inventory of activities. Interestingly, the category *Other PEL Initiatives* exceeds *Core Initiatives* by a ratio of over 8:1; this is consistent with the PEL program design, where community-specific activities are meant to be favoured over centrally developed programs.

Each of the four main role categories is further elaborated in the official PEL job description, yielding a total of 40 specific tasks. To streamline the format of the PEL survey, six key interrelated functions were abstracted from the full inventory of tasks. Although these functions do not necessarily capture everything a PEL might do, they help to offer a balanced picture of the priority activities and deliverables.

Table 3.3 PEL Activities by Focus and Platform, February and March 2010

	All PEL-Reported Activities	
	February (%)	March (%)
Activity Focus		
Primary Prevention	87.6	92.2
Screening	12.4	7.8
Total	100.0	100.0
Activity Platform		
Core Initiatives		
Tobacco Education and Action Module	3.8	2.9
Healthy Living Schools	6.7	3.9
Stop Smoking before Surgery	3.8	3.9
Social Media Working Group	1.9	1.0
Subtotal, Core Initiatives	16.2	11.7
Other PEL Initiatives		
Daycare/Primary/Elementary School	4.8	9.7
Secondary School	3.8	1.0
Postsecondary	4.8	6.8
Health Fair	8.6	8.7
Committees/Service Organizations/Professional Contacts	40.0	38.8
Other Community-Based	8.6	7.8
Media	3.8	2.9
Aboriginal/Cultural Specific	9.5	12.6
Subtotal, Other Initiatives	83.8	88.3
Total	100.0	100.0

Priority PEL Functions

The priority functions abstracted from the official job description are briefly described below, with some pertinent commentary offered by individual PELs.

1 **Networking.** This is perhaps the most fundamental aspect of PEL work, a prerequisite for most of their other assignments. It entails keeping up to date on the cancer prevention activities in a region, knowing the pertinent leaders, and making themselves known to the various groups. The task extends beyond information management to actively laying a foundation of trust and credibility that can lead to sharing success stories, identifying service gaps, receiving invitations to help, creating partnerships, etc. It was summed up as follows by one PEL: "You need to be a people person. You can't be afraid to cold call, or to talk with strangers or large groups. You need to be able to identify key people and key groups with which to collaborate in order to get the word out to the masses and make a difference." There is an unspoken recruitment "rule" in the PEL program, namely, to create early momentum whenever possible by hiring long-term residents who enjoy a good number of community connections in the target region.

2 **Building partnerships.** The formation of partnerships with key individuals, community groups, and institutions that share goals with BCCA Prevention Programs is facilitated through existing community connections and active networking. Partnerships usually entail "giving and getting." For example, public education sessions entail the PEL securing a platform to share the prevention message, and the community group or class receiving potentially lifesaving information. As well, helping another group or agency with one of its own action goals enables the PEL to extend his or her reach. The concept of partnership applies most powerfully to collaborative community action. The PEL may offer information on an issue, expertise in facilitating meetings, and/or the capability of representing a critical position to the media; resources brought to the table by the other partners make the whole effort stronger than the individual parts. While some partnerships seem logical, for instance between the PEL and tobacco counsellors from a health authority, many fruitful collaborations emerge within unlikely arenas. A PEL from the Vancouver area noted that some of their most successful

work was with local postsecondary institutions: "Many of them have student programming and events already taking place, and I have found that joining forces with them to get out our message of cancer prevention and screening to students has been success-ful. Many institutes have been receptive to the messaging, and have provided me with a perfect platform to do my work." The strong emphasis in the British Columbia program on partnerships is very consistent with the emerging literature supporting the importance of local, intersectoral, and other forms of cooperation in fulfilling the complex mandate of health education and promotion.

3 **Assessing community needs.** Knowing community needs related to cancer prevention is itself a complex function that could take all of the time available to a PEL. Inevitably, progress always must be pursued with incomplete information, but the goal remains to char-acterize community needs as accurately as possible. There are sev-eral avenues that can be involved, from the informal approach of "keeping one's ears open" (see Networking above) to more formal assessment tools administered to community leaders and members. In the best cases, it will also include a technical awareness of any cancer and risk-factor statistics that are available, as well as trends in the uptake of prevention interventions (e.g., screening rates). The intermediate outcome measure of a PEL's work involves asking whether the prevention initiatives result in behaviour change. By keeping their finger on the pulse of the community and providing programming that is tailored to the needs and desires of the popu-lation, PELs ensure that their efforts have as profound an impact as possible. As noted by one PEL: "Much of my work focuses on gain-ing a better understanding of my community, the barriers popu-lations face to experiencing good health and preventing chronic diseases. Meeting with members of my target populations has al-lowed me to gain a better understanding of their needs."

4 **Facilitating the implementation of community action plans.** Net-working with, and helping out with the plans of, local groups is already a way to move community action forward, but formal co-alitions and committee-based networks can "multiply the lever-age." This allows bigger objectives to be achieved, such as building a walking trail, launching a community garden, or sponsoring an anti-tobacco billboard. Given the extensive time commitment re-quired to participate in and organize such activities (particularly in the beginning stages), most PELs need to gauge where their

attention and skills are best used to facilitate the planning process and advance the agenda. One PEL described this type of work in the following way: "I assist by facilitating connections between individuals or groups, by providing them with information about each other, and possibly through introducing them to each other, in person or by phone or e-mail. I sometimes will co-lead groups or otherwise become involved at a leadership and/or committee level to help with getting plans started and implemented."

5 **Facilitating the implementation of the public education component of BCCA Prevention Programs.** Being informed is usually a prerequisite to making healthy lifestyle improvements. This applies equally to individuals who are at risk and to leaders who can make changes at an environmental level. Public education implies an audience; in the case of PELs, this usually is a community group or class, rather than the clinical model of counselling an individual or family. This is not to say that generating one-to-one encounters is excluded; such conversations can regularly arise, for example, around displays set up at community events. It is important to recognize that the goal of public health education does not just involve sharing information, but is aimed at creating participatory learning opportunities that will engage the audience and increase the possibility of application and change. A PEL recalled the following vignette: "One grade 3/4 class spontaneously took over a tobacco education time. Students jumped from topic to topic with all the energy and predictability of a dog's Kong toy. In the end, all the information I intended to present was covered completely by the children, with only minimal comments from me." PELs also play a key role in educating and informing their peers, such as other community organizers. One PEL noted that, since they are working for a taxpayer-funded organization, advocacy directed at government cannot be a focus of their efforts. However, it is still possible to operate in such situations by making a "shift from advocacy to an education component that relies on evidence-based information, in the hope that the steering committee as a group can make decisions based on such input; this allows me to indirectly play a role that informs the [advocacy] outcome."

6 **Making recommendations for cancer control policy.** This is a complex arena, one that can call on the PEL to act both locally and regionally. One example involved a PEL working at both of these levels in tobacco control. She made a presentation to a major retailer in the community aimed at reinforcing the importance of a policy

Figure 3.3. PEL Priorities.

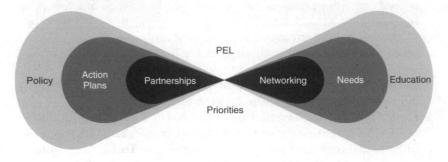

to not sell cigarettes in its pharmacy. As well, there were talks with the health authority leadership in the region to promote smoking restrictions on all health authority property; although this was already the official policy of the health authority, many health units did not consistently enforce it. Another PEL reflected on the following pertinent activities: "I have been able to make specific recommendations for cancer control. For example, a trail project to encourage physical activity, as well as shade for sun safety, including shade in daycare centres and shading to be incorporated at a local heritage park. There is further work to do – in particular, policies about offering healthier food choices at recreation centres and public events."

It is clear from the preceding descriptions that these functions of the PELs overlap and interconnect in various ways, with building partnerships and networking lying at the heart of the complex of activities, followed by identifying and planning around community needs (see Figure 3.3). Special content areas or targets important to the CPE role will be described further before offering some examples of (1) community engagement and (2) programs conceived by PELs or other planners.

Secondary Prevention (Screening)

Secondary prevention activities – mostly entailing promotion and education with respect to screening for breast and cervix cancers and pre-cancers – are a recent emphasis in the PEL portfolio. Overall, the PELs report a very positive experience with this component of their mandate. Many survey respondents stated that screening on its own merit is an important addition to their work, enhanced by the fact that promotion of screening also leads to primary prevention opportunities. One of the respondents offered the following endorsement: "My cancer screening work with a multicultural society has led to other opportunities with their immigrant health networks, such as delivering workshops around healthy eating and physical activity." Some PELs consider screening discussions a great starting point for networking, as suggested by the following comment: "This activity blends nicely with our role, and serves to establish new and valuable contacts to leverage off for other initiatives." A key initial concern for some PELs was that this expansion of their portfolio would add to or otherwise complicate their workload. However, it has been generally found that the screening focus did not add inordinate demands and that it certainly did not detract from the primary prevention agenda.

Special Populations

Although there are PELs acting as "point persons" for special populations in the province, cultural sensitivity is an essential aspect of the work of every PEL. The population of British Columbia is ethnically diverse. In particular, there are substantial numbers of recent immigrants of Chinese or South Asian background, the two groups with a specially assigned PEL. Many PELs also work closely with Aboriginal communities, or are seeking to develop relationships with such groups; this is especially important in the Northern Health Authority, which serves a population that is approximately 17% of Aboriginal background.

As one PEL noted, "because cultures are so diverse, adapting to their sensitivities is absolutely necessary to having a lasting impact." With this in mind, some PELs have attended workshops and other training sessions to improve their cultural competency. In order to be culturally appropriate, it is important that the prevention resources be adapted to the group in question. For instance, smoking is very prevalent among recent immigrants from East Asia, while obesity is not very common. South Asians as a group smoke to a lesser extent than the general population, but have a greater issue with obesity. Resources tailored to the need profile are made available through PELs in the appropriate language(s). With respect to newcomers from East and South Asia, as well as other immigrant populations, it is beneficial to look for other strategic ways to "get the prevention word out." This can include working alongside agencies and societies dedicated to assisting immigrants and refugees.

Aboriginal populations also require careful input and leadership. All PELs have finished or are enrolled in an "Indigenous Cultural Competency Online Training Program." There are specific techniques that have been found to be generally more effective here also. For instance, it is usually best to build trust and otherwise form a strong relationship with First Nations communities before attempting to implement any programs. As summed up by one PEL: "It's about building relationships and getting to know and understand each other, and how to communicate with each other, so that we can work together collaboratively, effectively, and productively." The basic strategy entails networking over a long time, including attendance at community events, making contacts with local health care providers who can facilitate introductions to Aboriginal leaders, and partnering with other organizations involved with First Nations peoples. The goal is to ensure that the PEL is established as an accessible and reliable resource with respect to disease prevention.

When giving presentations or workshops, the strategy needs to be adapted to fit with the communication style that is familiar to a particular culture. For instance, storytelling is important for Aboriginal groups, an approach that could involve using personal anecdotes to illustrate a prevention message and allowing time for participants to share their own experiences. "Audience participation" was particularly cited by PELs as key to generating respectful and effective communication with First Nations and other Aboriginal communities.

Community Engagement

The ability to engage the community in meaningful ways is critical to the success of a CPE-like program. In British Columbia this includes the use of environmental scans and community needs assessments. These tools offer direction to the PEL regarding where to focus their efforts and which stakeholders and potential partner organizations need to be engaged.

In general, the knowledge and awareness derived from the environmental scans and needs assessments has been very helpful, enabling staff to transfer knowledge by providing suggestions to other stakeholders who work in the health care field. In this way, resources will not be duplicated and invested in similar efforts; instead, unique initiatives will be supported that can build on each other.

Building networks to create further opportunities for partnerships, promotion, and education has been invaluable for broadening the reach and depth of what BCCA Prevention Programs have been able to achieve in British Columbia. This approach has been particularly successful in reaching immigrant and other vulnerable populations, as described in the following examples.

The South Asian Community

An environmental scan and needs assessment that analysed issues relating to cancer prevention was completed for the South Asian population. Understanding the types of cancer that most affect the South Asian community as well as the pertinent socioeconomic determinants enabled PELs to create specific strategies to target this population. Based on the scan, an approach was created that identified specific venues to target education and promotion efforts. For example, understanding the reasons behind higher incidence of oral cancer led to presenting information on consumption of chewing tobacco and areca/betel nut.

The environmental scan was also the first step in building community relations. It helped identify the other stakeholders and community partners who needed to be engaged to optimize program implementation. Working closely with other partners has since ensured that the goals are consistently met while minimizing duplicated efforts and wasted community resources. An application of this approach involved finding relevant programs being run by community agencies and accessing their clientele in order to spread the cancer prevention message. This was pursued, for example, among a group of young women in the "Best for Babies" program run by the Community Services of Abbotsford, a city near Vancouver.

A further layer to the community assessment process was an increased awareness of the cultural and gender sensitivities that needed to be considered when creating resources, distributing information, or trying to engage the target audience. For example, understanding both cultural and gender concerns helped PELs create a strategy to target South Asian women and encourage them towards breast and cervical screening.

The Chinese Community

Through an environmental scan and needs assessment conducted within the Chinese population, sun safety was determined to be of minimal concern because this population already tended to be vigilant about it. Tobacco use, however, was relatively high; this observation held particularly

among males (including recent immigrants), as well as young adult fe-
males. These sorts of data allowed prevention messaging to be prioritized
and adapted. For instance, the information indicated that masculine im-
agery should definitely be part of graphics related to smoking cessation.

An additional opportunity that grew from initial community assessments and relationship-building was a partnership with the Chinese
Canadian Medical Society of British Columbia to create a Chinese language *Stop Smoking Before Surgery* rack card; the aim was to assist physicians in the education of Chinese clients about the impact of smoking
on surgery outcomes.

Another important outcome entailed BCCA Prevention Programs/
PELs being one of seven partners to create a calendar for local community gardens that are used and maintained by long-term residents
as well as by new immigrants to Canada. The content throughout the
calendar involved a combination of healthy lifestyle/cancer risk-factor
prevention information and gardening tips and facts. A template of the
calendar was created that could be shared as a resource with any stakeholder wanting to pursue a similar initiative.

The Developmentally Disabled

The initial partnership of the PEL program with *posAbilities*, an organization that supports individuals of all ages with developmental dis-
abilities, opened the door for further partnership opportunities. For
example, BCCA Prevention Programs/PELs was the only health organization to attend the staff picnic held by *posAbilities* in the summer,
specifically to distribute information and otherwise educate about sun
safety. Other initiatives have included:

- Creating and sharing information on the five cancer-specific risk factors on the internal Health and Wellness website of the organization
- Designing and delivering nutrition and healthy living presentations
  and workshops to 600 staff members at their training centre
- Consulting on efforts to create a "healthy living plan" template for
  their clients that will comprise themes such as weight management,
  activity/exercise, and nutrition.

Component Programs

The term "program" is used in various ways in health care and even
within this book. It is important to clarify definitions before exploring

the topic further. On the broadest scale, a health care program may be a system of projects or services intended to meet a public health need. An example of such usage is offered in the following definition in a 1995 Institute of Medicine publication: "A comprehensive school health program is an integrated set of planned, sequential, school-affiliated strategies, activities, and services designed to promote the optimal physical, emotional, social, and educational development of students." The PEL network itself may be construed as such a system.

It is common, however, for some of the component projects or services coordinated or provided by a PEL to also be referred to individually as a program. This sense is the one that applies in the present chapter. It seems reasonable to limit the term program to those PEL-led projects or services that play a recurring role in most regions of the province; in this way, a program would be distinguished from a one-time project or event. Finally, the component programs may themselves have multiple elements (e.g., see Healthy Living Schools below), each of which may also be informally referred to as a program.

Before examining component programs that relate to the PEL agenda, it is important to recall a point made in the introductory chapter. As significant as programs are to their work, the PELs do not primarily engage in a "program delivery" model where plans developed elsewhere are "imposed" on a community. One PEL reinforced this point in the following way: "I have never swooped into a community with a boxed program but have consulted with the community and provided support in helping them build the necessary capacity to move towards healthier living."

The quotation above underlines the importance of another PEL commitment: any centrally designed program is always tailored to the specific needs and desires of the community and to the specific context in which it is delivered. This commitment was highlighted by another comment in a PEL interview:

> [Educators] from a national, provincial, or regional agency should shape any concept from a central program around the uniqueness of their region by adapting it to specific needs. This is especially noticeable when working with Aboriginal communities; they do not like to focus on disease, so I shift the cancer prevention message to a healthy lifestyles message. That is an area of concern, especially for new educators: achieving the balance between core programs and the individuality of their community.

Province-wide Prevention Programs

As described earlier, each PEL is responsible for mobilizing and coordinating strategies for action in cancer control within their community or region. Sometimes the connection is more of a support and enhancement role, such as increasing awareness of and participation in the Cervical Cancer Screening and Screening Mammography Programs (see the related section above).

In addition to various interagency collaborative projects and locally developed initiatives (see below), there are a number of province-wide prevention programs that are implemented regionally by the PELs – generally with the expectation that they will be customized as appropriate to align them with community needs. In some cases, the programs were developed by a committee made up of PEL members. Some of these are outlined briefly below.

HEALTHY LIVING SCHOOLS
The Healthy Living Schools Program was designed to assist schools in their health promotion efforts, specifically addressing tobacco cessation, sun safety, diet, and physical activity. Schools that fulfil certain prevention education standards are encouraged to register as a Healthy Living School in order to receive certification and specific materials and other resources to support further health promotion activities. There are currently over 700 schools registered in the program.

The PELs seek to encourage and support educators, notably by offering tangible services. Some of the ways that healthy living messages are reinforced include:

- Sports workshops
- Health fairs
- Educator mentorship
- Sun safety lessons
- Contests with small prizes for health-related activities
- Walking programs
- Web-based resources directed at students

There is a parallel program that recognizes preschool and daycare facilities in British Columbia that have instituted measures to help protect children from harmful exposure to the sun. "Sun Safe Facility" certificates are issued to daycare centres and preschools that meet essential sun safely requirements. These are facilities that have sufficient shade to allow all of their young children to be out of doors and yet remain in the shade as appropriate, and especially at times of peak sun exposure; in addition, they maintain a policy that hats are mandatory on field trips. So far, more than 1,700 daycares have been certified under the program.

WEBSITE HI5LIVING.ORG – GRADUATION TRANSITIONS
The British Columbia Ministry of Education's Graduation Transitions program is intended to prepare students for a successful transition to life after secondary school. It consists of three main components: work experience/community service, development of personal and career goals, and developing and maintaining a personal health plan. Hi5living, which is in the final stage of development, is intended to aid educators with the latter component. The program includes a cancer prevention quiz, strategies for lifestyle change, and action planning for good health that is related to reducing the risk of cancer. The associated web resource, www.hi5living.org, was developed with the assistance of teachers and school counsellors; it is tailored to those in the 15 to 18 year age group, but it has been found useful by others outside of the school system such as employers.

TOBACCO EDUCATION AND ACTION MODULE (TEAM)
The Tobacco Education and Action Module (TEAM) is a smoking cessation skills acquisition program designed to be used by facilitators outside of the health care professions, including teachers, counsellors, social workers, and others in contact with youth who smoke. The program teaches skills for communicating with a tobacco user, such as reflective listening and the creation of learning experiences. TEAM also provides aids for quitting, drawing from current research on tobacco cessation. The PELs offer the training module to community groups, schools, and others interested in tobacco education.

Individual PEL Initiatives

It is central to the PEL mandate to match initiatives to the needs of local citizens. This orientation has sparked the development of a number of creative programs in different parts of the province. The examples that follow represent innovations that have taken on the character of a recurring program, or have the potential to do so. It is also possible that the programs could be adapted in other areas of British Columbia, and even become instituted as a province-wide mandate.

PINK PARTIES

To increase awareness about the importance of regular mammograms in detecting breast cancer, one PEL in northern British Columbia started to provide "Pink Parties." These female-specific health initiatives involve displays and talks about women's health issues, with door prizes donated by local businesses. The parties often have a whimsical element, for example, "dry t-shirt" contests and outrageous pink costumes.

One challenge has been noted: "There has been difficulty in obtaining mammogram appointments at or near the time of the Pink Party. At one event, we had approximately 40 women enthusiastic about getting a mammogram. Six months later when we were able to book appointments, only 4 women attended – a 90% decrease in possible mammograms." The PEL went on to acknowledge that this problem has been solved simply by planning the parties around the time when the B.C. Cancer Agency mobile mammogram service will be in the community, resulting in a higher uptake rate.

CAFETERIA MAKEOVER

Following a presentation at the local school district, a PEL was approached by an enthusiastic new teacher who wanted advice on reopening the school cafeteria with healthier meal options; furthermore, the cafeteria was to be run by the students themselves. By helping the teacher brainstorm, reviewing her business plan, and connecting her with others for support, the PEL was instrumental in the new cafeteria launch, which was attended by local media. The "payoff" from such a project can be substantial; not only do students eat healthier, but many learn to cook, gain other valuable life skills, and generally grow in self-confidence.

ISLAND FITNESS CHALLENGE

An intercommunity Fitness Challenge was an example of the communication and partnership between neighbouring PELs. This program challenged residents of two communities to sign up and track their fitness-related efforts over a six-week period in January and February. Participants recorded the number of kilometres they logged each day, using a chart to translate common activities into kilometres. The program was facilitated through a local gym in each community, which also organized free weekly group activities. Overall, more than 500 individuals participated, with approximately 150,000 "kilometre equivalents" logged. At the end of the six weeks, the group from the winning community was awarded the privilege of directing half of the program registration fees from the opposing community to a local charity of their choice.

Organizational Success Factors

The creation of innovative component programs as described in the previous section already represents evidence of progress. But there are other ways to mark success in the Prevention Educational Leader strategy in British Columbia. Endorsement of the overall system and effort by an external body in charge of standards, auditing, or award-granting is of course very encouraging. As noted at the beginning of this chapter, the PEL program has been so recognized, with a major award being received in 2007.

A Canadian Community of Practice specific to this field has been established. It brings together the leaders of the provincial cancer programs with the goal of sharing best practices in cancer prevention delivery and evaluation. The development of a set of national standards for cancer agency prevention programs has been an important step in establishing more robust approaches to program evaluation. The standards have been categorized into three checklists that allow an agency to mark its progress from bronze to silver to gold recognition. Although it is not specific to the PEL strategy, the fact that the checklist for bronze recognition has been fulfilled by BCCA Prevention Programs is encouraging. The steps that need to be taken to move to the silver level were identified in a 2010–2013 strategic plan (see below, in the section Organizational Challenges).

Whatever else may be measured, it is relevant to point to the sense of satisfaction and progress expressed by various PELs. One PEL noted that every time she was asked to participate in a community workshop or project it felt as if her role in the community "was being viewed as an asset." Likewise, another PEL expressed job satisfaction as follows: "I enjoy making a difference. I have always wanted to work in a role where I can feel good about impacting the community positively. To me, at the end of the day, I need to know that all the time away from my

family was spent in education and development of the community."
Sometimes the "wins" experienced and expressed by PELs are more
focused; for example: "I have been able to alleviate some fears women
have concerning having mammograms and pap smears." Others stress
a broader sense of being appreciated by the people they serve: "By having a local PEL, they are seeing that they are being invested in as a community...that British Columbia cares about them, no matter how far
they are from the big cities."

Evaluation, however, ultimately should move beyond the global and
anecdotal to the specific and quantitative. The lack of robust evaluation
was a general concern expressed by the PELs, and this issue will be explored further in chapter 12. For the moment, it will suffice to review
how success is currently measured in the PEL program, and identify
factors that may have contributed to a sense of progress. Further analysis of important program elements will also be featured in Part C of the
book.

Evaluation Approaches

There are a number of component programs that generate quantitative
feedback for PELs. This includes the absolute number of screening encounters completed within a geographic area, and registrations of local
schools, daycares, and preschools under the Healthy Living Schools or
Sun Safe Facilities umbrellas. Less formal feedback is received through
interactions with community members at events, but at present no regular, formal evaluation forms are filled out by participants after events,
and there are no before-and-after surveys related to prevention knowledge, intentions, etc. However, the intent is to develop such a continuing evaluation process.

In discussing the various categories of program evaluation, one PEL
talked about the importance of qualitative feedback: "It serves the
funders very well to have the quantitative data, but they often miss
the importance of the qualitative data, and how it changes people and
their perspectives. For any of this work to make a real impact, we have
to be aware of the difference that it is making in the life of a person, a
whole person. This is not an either/or situation, but a recognition of the
equal value [of qualitative and quantitative evaluation]." Having said
this, it will become apparent to readers and reviewers of this book that,
with the exception of the North Karelia project in Finland, evaluation
remains a "weak link" in CPE-type strategies.

Regional Supervision

The addition of an administrator for the Northern Region has been considered a success. From an administrative perspective, it reduces the approval cycle for specific projects, media requests, and so on. The regional office is also a depot for materials, which are now positioned closer to many PELs. The process is still being refined; one PEL from northern British Columbia noted that there are still a number of requests that need to be approved at the provincial level, which has necessitated conversations with two levels of supervisors.

The Northern Region administrator acknowledged in an interview that there were obstacles in the first year of the expanded northern program, including finding and establishing a "bricks and mortar" office space, mapping out meeting times, and developing goals. But there have already been a number of positive developments. The first 2 years have seen the number of PELs in the region increase from three to ten, resulting in a proportionate jump in capacity-building and prevention activities in the associated communities.

PEL Working Groups

Although the PELs are largely focused on programs and other activities developed within their own regions, work has sometimes been pursued that is aimed at improving the overall PEL program or otherwise benefiting the province as a whole. This has included investigations of topics such as the social determinants of health and Aboriginal health. Occasionally, working groups led by veteran PELs explore or help to implement a specific area of prevention work. Two notable examples are the TEAM (Tobacco Education and Action Module) builders and a group looking at the prevention possibilities related to social media. One PEL summed up these sorts of initiatives as follows: "I think forming subcommittees for a specific topic is a good way to get PELs interacting and engaging across the province."

Mandate Expanded to Include Screening

The addition of screening to the mandate of PELs can be seen in part as a "bottom-up" development. On one hand, some PELs note that they were already providing screening information, responding to the strong desire expressed by community members for such services. On the other, the screening program managers recognized that PELs had the skills and proximity to enhance screening uptake in disadvantaged communities. With their expanded mandate, PELs can dedicate time and resources to the promotion of screening as time and opportunity allows. This serves as an example of how community engagement can help to drive policy and priorities at the provincial level. As noted earlier, the addition of screening to the PEL agenda has created a net gain: "I have found that screening does not detract from my primary prevention role but instead it can actually 'open doors' as a first point of conversation in outlying and remote communities."

Organizational Challenges

Time ... Not on One's Side

The reality of large geographical areas and/or populations, combined with part-time hours, makes it unsurprising that limited time is the challenge most often mentioned by PELs. The simplest ways to remedy this would be to increase the amount of overall working time per PEL, decrease the time spent on non-core activities, or hire additional PELs – the latter plan ultimately allowing for a smaller territory and population to be assigned. All of these potential solutions involve budgetary considerations.

The surveys of PELs indicated that any approaches to streamlining administrative requirements would be welcomed by them, and would be a benefit to the program as a whole. Increasing the number of regional administrators may help to reduce the administrative load the PELs currently carry, but at a potential cost of fewer "boots on the ground" in the community. The need for PELs to check with the client, BCCA Prevention Programs, before pursuing certain parts of their assignment may mean some efficiency gaps; although it is true that PELs work more independently than most employees, it is not clear whether they have more or less practical autonomy than do "official" leaders and spokespeople. The rationale for continuing institutional oversight is that the B.C. Cancer Agency is an evidence-driven organization, with high standards regarding what constitutes reliable data. PELs, in contrast, come from a wide variety of educational backgrounds that may not have provided the tools for rigorous assessment of evidence. This is particularly an issue in the area of environmental carcinogens, where the general public tends to focus on the "last headline" and broad, ill-defined worries. In contrast, the B.C. Cancer Agency focuses on International Agency for Research on Cancer (IARC) class 1 and 2A carcinogens, as defined and updated by a continuing review of the scientific evidence.

As suggested earlier in the Qualifications section, the contract employment arrangement with some PELs in British Columbia undoubtedly has certain advantages, but it is in fact a unique paradigm – all of the other model programs in the world investigated for this book are based on full-time educators or coordinators hired as regular employees. Some PELs have developed specific "game plans" in an effort to make the most of their part-time assignments. One PEL chose to spend their first year focusing on two specific areas of expertise, nutrition and sun safety. In the following year, being more comfortable in the role, that PEL expanded their focus in the direction of Aboriginal health. On one hand, a periodic shift in focus was one way to embrace and express their generalist mandate; on the other hand, maintaining a specific focus at any one time prevented a dilution of effectiveness, allowing them to do fewer things better.

Organizational Priority and Media Exposure

There are many messages and messengers in the public realm related to health care in general and prevention in particular. This creates synergies within the work of PELs when, for instance, the prevention messages of different organizations overlap. However, there can also be a sense of competing for attention in the midst of a busy, noisy arena. Increasing public awareness of the PEL program would enhance the credibility of PELs, facilitating their admittance to certain circles of influence; it would also increase the odds of community groups and health care professionals seeking them out. Media exposure is itself a paradigm faced with accelerating change; the working group addressing the role of social media in the PEL task is one way the program is seeking to get "ahead of the curve."

Apart from external obstacles and opportunities, there is the ongoing challenge of how prevention in general and the PELs in particular are positioned in the overall world of the British Columbia Cancer Agency. One PEL noted that funding for the Prevention Programs represents less than 0.3% of the total BCCA budget, with most of the rest going to chemotherapy and radiation therapy services in five regional cancer centres and in satellite chemotherapy clinics.

Areas of Growth and Improvement

Through strategic planning processes, the BCCA as a whole and the Prevention Programs area in particular look towards improvements in the future. The 2010–2013 plan related to prevention identified four activity objectives that, if fulfilled, would enable the overall program to be recognized as satisfying a "silver" standard according to the categories developed by a national Community of Practice for cancer prevention professionals (see Appendix II). The four objectives relate to:

- Engaging clinicians as advocates for primary prevention
- Providing skill development to communities, partner organizations, other provincial cancer agency staff, etc.
- Developing collaborative partnerships with cancer treatment and disease management organizations
- Monitoring behavioural risk factors for cancer prevention

The first two points in this list were rated as the highest priorities by PELs in their survey responses. The first matter, implementing interventions to increase engagement of primary care in the prevention task, could be particularly challenging for PELs. Such advances may need to be initially driven at other leadership levels in the BCCA or even the Provincial Health Services Authority, of which BCCA is but a part, and the five regional health authorities that deliver most general medical services. There is good evidence from the first case study, the North Karelia Project detailed in the next part of the book, that all health care platforms need to be committed to the prevention agenda, especially primary care providers. In Finland, the recruiting of physicians and other clinicians to the cause likely happened more from "the top" rather than through "bottom-up" interventions from prevention workers in the field. There may be a place for "prevention detailing" or outreach/training visits by PELs to primary care clinics, but only with some contextual preparation led at other planning levels in the province. In other words, it is unlikely that PELs would be enthusiastically received by physicians without some prior "buy-in" by the medical system.

Finally, the relatively low priority given by PELs to the fourth growth area, monitoring behavioural risk factors, reflects the importance of the prioritized areas from the perspective of population health, but also may suggest the need for a greater understanding of the importance of evaluation data, a topic that will be reviewed further in chapter 12.

Sources and Further Reading

BCCA information on the real facts about skin cancer. Available at www.sun-tips.ca (accessed 15 April 2010).

British Columbia Cancer Agency Strategic Plan. Updated October 2006. Available at www.bccancer.bc.ca/NR/rdonlyres/1C2F0481-8451-4CF8-82EC-0294BB2D492B/19827/BCCA_Strategic_Plan_Updated_Oct06.pdf (accessed 23 January 2010).

Cancer Prevention Brochures (English, Punjabi, Chinese). Available at http://www.bccancer.bc.ca/PPI/Prevention/about/PreventionProgramsPublications.htm (accessed 15 April 2010).

Cancer Research UK. Statistics on the risk of developing cancer. Available at http://info.cancerresearchuk.org/cancerstats/incidence/risk/ (accessed 23 January 2010).

Carlow DR. The British Columbia Cancer Agency: a comprehensive and integrated system of cancer control. Hosp Q. 2000;3(3):31–45. Medline:11494610

Healthy Living Challenge. Available at www.hi5living.org (accessed 15 April 2010).

Healthy Living Schools Initiative. Available at http://www.bccancer.bc.ca/PPI/Prevention/about/programs/schools.htm (accessed 8 February 2010).

Jones J, Barry MM. Exploring the relationship between synergy and partnership functioning factors in health promotion partnerships. Health Promot Int. 2011;26(4):408–20. http://dx.doi.org/10.1093/heapro/dar002. Medline:21330307

PART B

Other Models of Community-Based Prevention Educators

4 Identifying Models of Prevention Coordination in the Community

There are many examples and categories of community-based prevention efforts throughout the world. Paring down the total list of programs depends on abstracting an initial, basic paradigm of the CPE position as it is found in British Columbia.

CPE Definition as a Selection Grid

A working definition of a community-based prevention educator was proposed in the preceding chapter of the book:

> A professional leader coordinating community-based efforts to reduce the common risk factors and/or progression of cancer and other chronic disease in a defined population.

This definition may be unpacked in terms of four fundamental dimensions, specifically related to the category, scope, manner, and purpose of the leadership involved. Some other characteristics may be implied by the definition of a CPE, but the following dimensions are intrinsic to it. Note that it is important to delineate each dimension both by what it means and by what it does not mean.

Dimension 1. Professional Leadership
The CPE works as a paid consultant within a broad arena of health care planning and coordination; they typically have some form of advanced training in an allied field. In contrast, there are many programs in the world that entail recruiting and mobilizing lay volunteers to facilitate a specific kind of health care service delivery for people in a

Figure 4.1. Four Dimensions of CPE Definition.

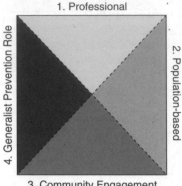

local area; this role has many titles, but the most common one is "community health worker." Although some perks and even a modest stipend may be involved with this role, the position of a lay worker is quite distinguishable from the fully remunerated professional leadership offered by a CPE.

Dimension 2. Defined Population Target

The word "community" is notoriously varied in its meaning in the literature and in practice, and "community-based" is not much better. This is why it may be better to think of CPEs in terms of a population, or being population-based. There are two connotations attached to this idea: first, a population represents the scope of practice, rather than individuals or households; and, second, the targeted population is clearly defined or limited, usually by geography and sometimes also by ethnocultural group. Thus, the work of the CPE is distinguished from clinical prevention, where the focus is one-to-one encounters (and sometimes families or a small, unrelated group of people). Putting it differently, CPEs are occupied with a type of public health function, rather than with the activities usually associated with primary care of individual clients. Again, the focus of the CPE is generally the whole population (however defined) and all levels and settings in society, although specific efforts tailored to substantial sub-groups may be part of the strategy.

Dimension 3. Community Engagement

The word "educator" in the title CPE points to a stance towards the community that is responsive rather than directive. In other words, CPEs tend to work in an organic, "bottom-up" manner that at least takes the health needs of a community into consideration, and generally goes further by devising solutions in collaboration with community members and/or relevant agencies serving the community. This means that CPEs are geared primarily to coordinating a conversation about strategies for health, rather than coordinating service delivery per se. It is not typical for CPEs to administrate programs in a "top-down" way, to be the local agent of a national campaign, or the like. If specific programs are promoted by a CPE, this would generally entail some adaptation to the population and "culture" of the target community.

Dimension 4. Generalist Prevention Role

The vocabulary related to "prevention" also represents a large and variable domain. The best way to distinguish different types of prevention is to ask: what is being prevented? For CPEs, the key target is the common behavioural risk factors of cancer and other chronic disease. Notably, this includes smoking, physical inactivity, and unhealthy eating (especially overnutrition leading to overweight), as well as certain ecological influences on the behavioural choices of individuals. Sun protection and reducing exposure to environmental agents are additional concerns specific to cancer. The CPE is not a specialist in terms of one risk factor or one strategy, but enjoys a generalist prevention role. This extends beyond the primary prevention arena to embrace certain secondary prevention efforts, such as screening for disease precursors. There are still some limits on the scope of practice: supporting medical treatment to avoid disease progression or co-morbidities is generally not on the agenda.

Locating and Selecting Cases to Study

Each of the preceding dimensions will be explored in more detail in later chapters. For now, it is enough to know that the four dimensions acted as a guide to choosing the global comparators to be described in this part of the book. The process for selecting cases is outlined below.

First, the potential inventory of cases was assembled from three main sources:

- General review of biomedical databases (e.g., PubMed) and grey literature, with key search terms such as "community prevention educator" and variants
- Targeted review of community-based prevention programs in jurisdictions comparable to British Columbia
- Referrals from case study interviewees and other key informants

The approach involved identifying a large enough number of pertinent cases to increase the confidence in any principles that were ultimately abstracted. To this end, what is known as "replication logic" rather than "sampling logic" was applied; in other words, a case was added to the inventory not first to look for variation across a wide range of programs, but instead with the goal of finding similar results (i.e., replication) across one or more domains of interest. In this type of research, replication over several cases is designed to maximize assurance in the final results.

Selection Criteria

How was the replication of results achieved? There were several qualifications of community prevention educators that were considered as a guide, but not ultimately adopted as a basis for selecting cases. For instance, no distinction was made between short-term programs (i.e., pilots or studies or campaigns) and those established over the long term. Although sustainability is always a concern, it was still thought to be important to derive lessons from experiences that lasted only months rather than many years. The idea was that if a program (no matter how long it functioned) had certain compelling qualities, then it could be abstracted and used to inform a program with a longer lifespan. Naturally, if a shorter program is selected as a case, any evidence of gaps leading to a lack of sustainability would be one area of learning not to be missed.

Similarly, a case study was not selected based on sponsorship. Although a core government program (or a quasi-government effort led by an organization such as a cancer agency) may have more likelihood of sustained funding and leadership, non-governmental community prevention efforts will sometimes generate valuable lessons to help official policymakers.

Finally, the level of success enjoyed by a program did not automatically lead to inclusion or exclusion as a case study. The fact is that lessons learned from a "failed" experiment can sometimes be the most valuable of all.

What were the important positive selection criteria?

Apart from the commonly desired goal of drawing on examples with geographical diversity, it seemed reasonable that the highest utility would come from developing case studies where the program came *closest to matching the CPE organizational and content patterns*. Practically, this meant that the types of leadership positions to be described and analysed in the case must, as a starting point, incorporate a majority of the four defining dimensions summarized above. This approach had immediate value as a rule of thumb with respect to both exclusions and inclusions. As will be seen below, understanding what not to include is just as important as identifying the eventual inventory of case studies pursued.

Exclusionary Power

For example, the substantial literature devoted to lay community health workers was found not to be directly pertinent, because that type of position usually does not match up well with the CPE dimensions. One well-known instance of community health workers is found in communities along the United States–Mexico border. The *Salud para su Corazon* (Health for Your Heart) intervention program involves *promotores de salud* ("health promoters"), understood to be equivalent to what other programs call community health workers. The *promotores* (or female *promotoras*) encourage healthy nutrition and physical activity in Hispanic communities, with the aim of reducing the disproportionate burden of cardiovascular disease (CVD) among this group. *Promotores* work as part of a larger team consisting of medical care providers and support staff, diabetes educators, and administrators. They recruit people to meet with physicians, helping new clients to navigate the medical system, while at the same time presenting information to individuals and small groups on the specific factors and lifestyle changes that are related to the risk of CVD.

Such lay worker programs do not map directly onto the CPE position. The CPE generally comes with a higher level of training and a broader scope of professional responsibility, with commensurate remuneration. This does not mean that the two program types do not demonstrate overlaps. Indeed, a direct connection may be found with CPE-type scenarios where one of the emergent tasks is to create and supervise a network of community health workers. In other words, community health workers can be a way in which prevention educators accomplish their purpose. As well, *promotores* work in an organizational context (the so-called Community Health Center) that corporately delivers services similar to the CPEs; these include public relations and media efforts, community outreach events, and developing partnerships with health departments, schools, and other organizations.

Other programs approximated the CPE model, but were still eliminated because of alternatives in the list that demonstrated a superior fit. An example would be tobacco control officers who are hired in many higher income countries to work on a regionalized basis. The main features of this model that distinguish it from the CPE program are the focus on a single risk factor rather than a more generalist, comprehensive agenda, and the fact that it tends to have a "top down," program-delivery flavour. Such an approach does in fact exist in British Columbia itself, the well-respected Regional Tobacco Reduction Officers. Similar to the situation found with lay community health workers, these regional risk factor-specific officers ultimately are different from CPEs, although they still represent potential partners in fulfilling the goals of a more general prevention approach. Another example of regional allies would be the nutrition education staff hired by health authorities; although still working on a more limited risk factor agenda, these leaders do tend to enjoy some freedom in the development of strategies, including the potential for collaboration with other organizational actors in the arena of prevention of chronic disease.

A final example of a "close but not quite" program is the New Zealand initiative with the title "A Pilot Programme for Lifestyle and Exercise," or APPLE. This project was a community-based obesity prevention initiative located in primary schools in the communities of Otago and Dunedin. The 2-year program focused on promoting physical activity and nutrition in order to improve short-term and long-term health outcomes; a notable aim was to stem the progression of childhood obesity. It did not qualify as a case study for the present purpose because it only focused on one setting and age group in society and there was only modest pursuit of opportunities for community engagement.

Inclusionary Power

The cases finally identified as most useful to study are outlined in Table 4.1, with the applicable CPE dimensions indicated.

The five programs that will be developed as case studies in the ensuing chapters are distinguished by matching the majority, and usually all four, of the CPE dimensions. Two of them are based in the United States,

Table 4.1 Case Studies Compared on CPE Dimensions

Position Title (Program Name)	Jurisdiction	Dimensions*			
		I	II	III	IV
Field Office Staff Team (North Karelia Project)	Finland	•	•	•	•
Health Promotion Officers (Action Cancer)	Northern Ireland	•	•		•
Cancer Control Specialists / Extension Agents (KCP / HEEL)	Kentucky	•	•	•	•
Supervisor of Community Health Ambassadors (CHA Program)	North Carolina	•	•		•
Health Promotion Coordinators (Regional Health Authorities)	Manitoba	•	•	•	•
Example Exclusions					
Promotores (Salud Para Su Corazón)	Mexico–U.S. border	•	•		•
Activity Coordinators (School-based) (A Pilot Programme for Lifestyle and Exercise)	New Zealand (Otago + Dunedin)				•

*I = Professional Leadership; II = Defined Population Target; III = Community Engagement; IV = Generalist Prevention Role a testament to that country's commitment to large-scale public health initiatives. The oldest (and most famous) program on the list is the one from Finland, which originated with a project in the 1970s in the region known as North Karelia. In recent decades, the United Kingdom has emerged as a leader in public health innovation, so it is not surprising to find a case originating there, specifically from Northern Ireland. Finally, the Canadian province of Manitoba offered a helpful comparison with and counterpoint to the CPE program developed in British Columbia.

Method and Value of Case Study Research

Investigators have used the case study research approach for many decades across a variety of disciplines. It is a qualitative research method that is especially employed in the social sciences. Concerns have been expressed about it, mostly related to the reliability and generalizability of results derived from a small number of cases.

Researcher R.K. Yin offered the following characterization of case studies in a seminal textbook first published 25 years ago: "an empirical inquiry that investigates a contemporary phenomenon within its real-life context." For the present purpose, the phenomenon in focus is a program of prevention educators focused on cancer or broader chronic disease; the context is the particular jurisdiction (and population) in which the program operates.

In addition to selecting the cases, Yin and other authorities have laid out several basic steps that enter into the classic case study approach:

- Define the purpose of the project and the pertinent research questions
- Determine the information-gathering plan
- Collect the information
- Evaluate/analyse the information
- Summarize relevant results, including patterns and outliers

The way in which these steps were applied in the current project is summarized below.

Research Questions

The purpose of the case study component of this book was to underline and characterize the valuable aspects of a program such as the Community-Based Prevention Educators in British Columbia and to gain some insight about their generalizability for other jurisdictions. As stated earlier, the target audience is policy-planners seeking to establish (or refine) a chronic disease prevention program. This naturally generated three overarching research questions to be posed within each case study:

1 What are the parallels with the context and content of the prevention educator program?
2 What are the contrasts?
3 What insights may be gleaned about the value and character of a prevention educator program similar to the one in British Columbia?

Information Collection and Analysis

The basic information on the programs of interest and specific reflections on the research questions were assembled through two well-travelled routes: (a) a literature review guided by consulting health care databases combined with general Internet searching for pertinent grey literature; and (b) interviews with program leaders and other key informants. The interview format was semi-structured; the framework included inquiries serving the main research directions listed above, but allowed for the pursuit of side trails unique to the case at hand. This approach permitted flexibility concerning the direction of the conversation, while maintaining the potential for comparability between programs during the evaluation and analysis phase. Interview notes were taken by at least two researchers to maximize completeness and reliability.

As will become evident in the chapters to follow, there was a great deal of richness in the case studies, with many insights for policy-makers planning to adopt or adapt a CPE-type program in their jurisdiction.

Sources and Further Reading

Balcázar H, Alvarado M, Cantu F, et al. A promotora de salud model for addressing cardiovascular disease risk factors in the US-Mexico border region. Prev Chronic Dis. 2009;6(1):A02. Medline:19080008

McAuley KA, Taylor RW, Farmer VL, et al. Economic evaluation of a community-based obesity prevention program in children: the APPLE project. Obesity (Silver Spring). 2010;18(1):131–6. http://dx.doi.org/10.1038/oby.2009.148. Medline:19444231

Yin RK. *Case Study Research: Design and Methods*. 4th ed. Thousand Oaks, CA: Sage Publications; 2009.

5 North Karelia: Field Office Staff

There were many components to the North Karelia Project, including well-accepted health promotion activities that were pursued very vigorously, as well as a few notable innovations. For instance, a weekly television program was aired featuring 10 North Karelians who regularly had their blood pressure and other risk factors measured as they pursued different health improvement strategies. The series was very popular all over Finland, with various versions of the show running for 15 years. The director of the North Karelia Project recalls being stopped by strangers around the country and being asked if such and such a guest had managed to stop smoking ... He may well have used such opportunities to "get the word out" about all of the other creative work going on behind the scenes, including the hypertension screening efforts and related registry, the healthy cooking clubs, the training of lay health leaders, the negotiations with dairy producers to get low-fat products onto store shelves. The television show, although it had a high profile, was really only one piece of a much larger picture.

This case study focuses on specific aspects of the North Karelia Project, the famous and influential community-wide cardiovascular health program in Finland. As suggested above, the project was in some respects far ahead of its time, anticipating the power and popularity of today's "reality TV" phenomenon. In other ways, it fully reflected its time, embracing an emerging prevention culture that was committed to pursuing community-wide initiatives and other core expressions of health promotion. Continuing to make North Karelia a focus might be considered inappropriate, since the program in that province was in fact adopted as a national initiative and multiplied to other parts of

Figure 5.1. Map of North Karelia.

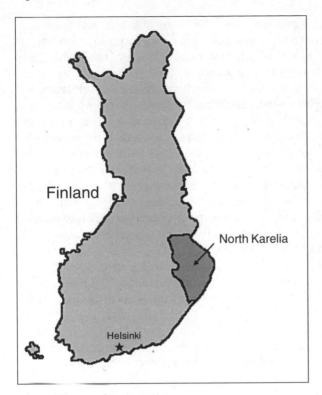

the country only a few years after its launch in the 1970s. However, the reporting and analysis over the ensuing decades have continued to highlight the work in North Karelia, even to this day, when the intensive "demonstration project" aspect of the program has come to an end and the principles and practices have been woven into the fabric of public health across the country. In fact, the pioneering director of the effort, Professor Pekka Puska, has published almost 400 journal articles to date, over half of which deal in some way with the North Karelia Project itself or its extension to other parts of Finland.

A Program for the World

Studies comparing countries in the 1950s and 60s showed that coronary heart disease mortality rates among Finnish men were among the highest in the world, and North Karelia's rate was 40% higher than the national one, even though its economy was dominated by physically active jobs such as logging and farming. However, while strenuous work kept the Finns relatively slim, they still enjoyed their butter, whole milk, sausage, salt, and cigarettes; conversely, fruits and vegetables were rarely on the menu. The region of North Karelia was also afflicted by poverty and other social issues; the deep roots of these problems may be partly found in the conflicts with the neighbouring Soviet Union during the Second World War, which eventually resulted in parts of the historic Karelian region being removed from Finnish jurisdiction. This challenging sociopolitical background helps to explain the 1972 petition sent by local leaders to secure government support in improving the health of the population.

In response to the original appeal, local and national authorities were mobilized, as well as experts from the World Health Organization (WHO). The North Karelia Project was designed from the beginning to:

- Implement comprehensive interventions
- Work through community organizations
- Facilitate grassroots participation from the target population
- Carry out full, continuous evaluation
- Provide a major demonstration program for national and international applications related to noncommunicable disease (NCD) prevention

These objectives appear to have been well met. For instance, in terms of the last point, the North Karelia Project (along with Finland as a whole) has strongly contributed to the WHO's European Countrywide Integrated Noncommunicable Disease Intervention (CINDI) program, and more recently to the Global Forum on NCD Prevention and Control. The CINDI program was developed in 1984 with the aim of creating and evaluating intervention strategies and methods for chronic disease prevention.

The Finnish CINDI Director is Professor Erkki Vartiainen, who also has been one of the chief leaders and researchers within the North Karelia Project. In order to augment the many published reports on the

North Karelia Project, an interview was conducted with Professor Vartiainen in March 2010. An MD and PhD, and currently assistant director general of the National Institute for Health and Welfare in Helsinki, Vartiainen started his career as a medical student attached to the North Karelia Project in 1976. Shortly after the interview with him, Professor Pekka Puska also generously made himself available to the authors, especially to reflect on how the educators and front-line staff had been organized to achieve the results seen in North Karelia. Dr Puska is currently the director general of the National Institute for Health and Welfare in Finland and president of the World Heart Foundation, as well as having several other international roles.

Strategic Processes and Solid Outcomes

The North Karelia Project was designed around the principles of health promotion. Classically, this means paying attention to all levels of change to promote health: individual healthy behaviours, community or environmental factors conducive to making healthy choices, and the broadest social determinants of health influenced by policies that generally fall outside of the sphere of health services. The project classified its comprehensive approach to risk factor change around six domains:

- Improved clinical preventive services to identify high-risk individuals and provide treatment
- Information to educate people about their health and how to maintain it
- Persuasion to motivate people towards healthy choices
- Training to increase skills of self-control, management of one's environment, and collaborative action to increase physical assets and social capital with the potential to benefit health
- Community organization to create social support and power for social action
- Environmental change to create opportunity and support for healthy actions and improvements in unfavourable conditions

According to Professor Vartiainen, the evaluation component of the North Karelia Project was also very robust from the start. Indeed, scientists were an intimate part of the project team, moving from village to village with other staff, gathering, analysing, and reporting data at every stage. The capacity to track process indicators, as well as the

Figure 5.2. Mortality Rates Due to Coronary Heart Disease: Males Aged 35–64, North Karelia and All of Finland, Age-Adjusted, 1969–2006.

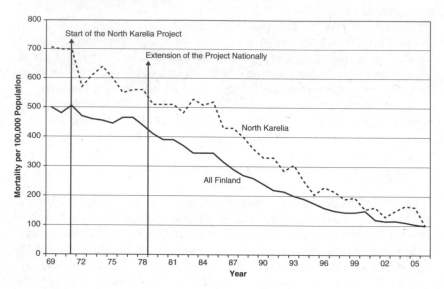

"harder" outcomes related to disease rates, likely represents one of the key engines of the project's success.

As suggested above, evaluation strategies and structures represent a key public health export from Finland to the rest of the world. It is no coincidence, for example, that the data centre for the WHO program known as MONICA (MONItor trends in CArdiovascular diseases) was established in the early 1980s in Helsinki, the capital of Finland. MONICA was supposed to help explain the diverse global trends in cardiovascular disease mortality. There were ultimately over 30 MONICA Collaborating Centres established in 21 countries, monitoring some 10 million men and women aged 25–64 years. A decade of data collection has been completed, and most of the main results have already been published. In a similar vein, the Chronic Disease Prevention Unit of Finland's newly formed National Institute for Health and Welfare continues to offer leadership in the noncommunicable disease data collection system used by CINDI countries (i.e., CINDI Health Monitor). The momentum for such intensive data collection and analysis may be ultimately traced to the oft-reported outcomes of the North Karelia

Project. There is an understandable desire to reproduce the positive results from what one commentator referred to as a "sweet spot" for public health studies.

The encouraging health trend in North Karelia was already evident
as early as 5 years after the launch of the project, and it has been steadily
confirmed in the decades since. As Figure 5.2 shows, CHD mortality
has dropped by approximately 80% in about 30 years. Analysis suggests that at least three quarters of the remarkable CHD mortality de-
cline seen among middle-aged men in particular may be attributed to
improvement in diet and decreases in smoking. The biological mark-
ers confirm this conclusion: serum cholesterol and blood pressure have
both greatly declined among men and women, although blood pressure has actually levelled off since 2002. The latter plateau may reflect
the countervailing force of increasing body-mass index in the population, which only serves to underline that, even in North Karelia, the
public health battle is never over. Indeed, across the whole country,
there is a new emphasis on tackling obesity, physical inactivity, and the
growing rate of type 2 diabetes.

A Reproducible Model?

A portion of the substantial commentary on North Karelia has been occupied with explaining why its approach has not been as effective in
other settings. This especially applies to the effort to change the diet of
a population in order to generate changes in the cardiovascular realm.
For instance, the Multiple Risk Factor Intervention Trial (MRFIT) of the
1970s did demonstrate a strong, linear connection between serum cholesterol and coronary heart disease (CHD) mortality, but was unable to
show an effect when either behavioural or biological risk factors were
reduced. MRFIT was a randomized primary prevention trial involving
12,866 high-risk men aged 35 to 57 years. Men were randomly assigned
either to a special intervention (SI) program consisting of stepped-care
treatment for hypertension, counselling for tobacco use, and dietary
advice for lowering blood cholesterol levels, or to their usual sources of
health care in the community (UC). Over an average follow-up period
of 7 years, risk factor levels declined in both groups, but to a greater degree for the SI group. However, mortality from CHD was 17.9 deaths
per 1,000 in the SI group and 19.3 per 1,000 in the UC group, a statisti-
cally non-significant difference; similarly, *total* mortality rates were 41.2
per 1,000 (SI) and 40.4 per 1,000 (UC).

The broader, community-based approaches launched in the 1980s in Stanford, Minnesota, and other U.S. regions also yielded unconvincing results. Despite this track record, comprehensive health promotion strategies at the population level have not been abandoned. For example, the general approach has been undergoing a renaissance in European centres, a development that is now spreading to other parts of the world. Operating under the heading EPODE (Ensemble, Prévenons L'Obésité des Enfants [Together Let's Prevent Childhood Obesity]), there have been encouraging outcomes reported in the region of France where it was pioneered; however, it is fair to say that the evaluation component of this model is still in its infancy.

Behind such efforts always lurks the question: What aspects of the North Karelia Project need to be reproduced to maximize the potential for reducing risk factors and, ultimately, reducing disease rates? Previous case studies have tried to identify missing dimensions in other programs that may account for the lack of positive results. The following insights have been proposed by Sara Kreindler of Manitoba, Canada, and other reviewers:

- The evaluation grids applied to the various projects have been quite heterogeneous, rarely matching the robustness of the North Karelia model.
- Some community-based efforts, while supposedly comprehensive and multicomponent, "may simply consist of the old mass-media approach in disguise" or otherwise depend too much on environmental interventions with too small a dose to create a significant effect.
- The unique features of the Karelian project have not been considered, including that it operated in an unhealthy region that was motivated to change and therefore *approached the government for help.* In contrast, the U.S. projects from the 1980s had a top-down design that was the opposite of the well-tested community development model where "trained facilitators follow the community's lead."

Professor Vartiainen provided a balancing perspective on the last point. It is not that experts have no role in motivating a community to change. If scientists had not first assembled and reported the alarming data on coronary heart disease rates in North Karelia, the original appeal for help might never have happened or been so compelling. However, Professor Vartiainen did agree that the intensive interaction of experts with the population was fundamental to the development, evaluation, and adjustment of ultimately successful community-based interventions. In short, credible scientific data was essential at every stage, as well as ongoing community dialogue and involvement.

The role of scientists on the team in North Karelia moves the discussion towards the main theme of the present case study, namely, understanding how all of the professional staff were organized and deployed in order to achieve such positive outcomes.

The Team and Its Activities

The staff of the North Karelia Project Field Office was carefully assembled. This characterization applied to different aspects of team-building – from basic capacity to skill sets to institutional supports (see Figure 5.3).

The main feature of the organization at the field level is that a *team* with various specializations was responsible for the whole region, rather than a series of generalists being assigned, for example, one to a village. According to Dr Puska, the field office team was always small, comprising a complement of about half a dozen members; according to needs and the budget available, it ranged as high as 10 people. Thus, on average the staff-to-population ratio was about 1 to 30,000 (based on a North Karelian population in the 1970s of approximately 180,000). This may be contrasted sharply with, for example, the ratio of Area Health Specialists in the California Diabetes Program; currently, five such staff people cover different regions within a state that has a total population of *37 million*.

While the field office team worked from a centralized location, there was also an attempt to localize efforts in a tangible way. For instance, a new office connected to the project was established in each of the 12 community health centres of North Karelia. Among other values, Dr Puska explained that this helped to mobilize local public health nurses and physicians, thereby multiplying the personnel beyond the field office staff. This approach was also consistent with the traditional orientation in Finnish society towards organizing at a municipal level.

What were the activities of the team? Generally, the efforts were directed to both individuals and the community as a whole. Initially, there was a big focus on control of hypertension. The nurses of the team managed a region-wide hypertension registry that was gradually populated with information derived through mass screening programs at country fairs, village markets, etc. Individuals with elevated blood pressure were referred to physicians and then monitored and prompted with

Figure 5.3. North Karelia Project: Oversight and Staff.

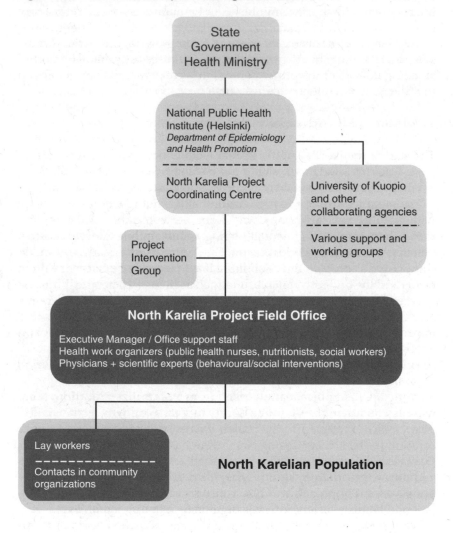

respect to medications and lifestyle modifications. Another program involving individual-level work was a based on a "quit and win" strategy where smokers entered a contest where prizes could be garnered in the event of proven cessation.

Team members consistently acted as communication agents throughout the community. This involved disseminating information on risk factors and prevention in various settings, from supermarkets to homes to clubs to community meetings. The campaign began with simple pamphlets offering heart-healthy eating suggestions and tips for smoking cessation, but later became more sophisticated. For instance, nutritionists on the team helped to run more intensive training courses and other community programs aimed at nutritious cooking and eating. Project staff organized over 300 "Parties of Long Life," where families gathered to try out new, healthier recipes and listen to lectures by Dr Puska and his colleagues. The field office was proactive about getting educational and inspirational stories into the formal media, and the North Karelia Project benefited to a great extent from journalists picking up on the good news independently. As a result, media coverage was extensive.

Another important information conduit involved community health education diffused through lay opinion leaders from formal and informal groups; public health nurses, physicians, and others connected to the team were involved with recruiting and training them. Forming partnerships with other health organizations, such as the Heart Association, was also critical to this endeavour. The sense of collaboration was very broad, multiplying the core project team many times over. Ultimately, thousands of ordinary citizens cooperated through small actions such as displaying a sticker or poster in their homes or workplaces. Regional pride was one of the emotional factors brought to bear, for example, through public signage reading "Do not smoke here – we are in the North Karelia Project." The team was responsible for researching and sourcing or creating these sorts of materials.

While the various individual and small group efforts continued, the focus was expanded to society as a whole. Two main community-wide goals were on the agenda of the North Karelia Project: to increase the availability of low-fat food to substitute for the saturated dairy/animal fat that dominated regional menus, and to introduce restrictions on smoking in indoor spaces such as restaurants. Different members of the project team were involved with direct and indirect advocacy for this type of environmental change. The direct approach involved sitting down with shop proprietors and the management of food processing plants in the area. The idea was to enlist cooperation in making healthier food options available to the population, including low-fat milk products. The indirect approach included team members fostering a sense of social action among lay opinion leaders to increase the pressure on decision-makers.

Finally, there were several examples of success achieved by Puska and colleagues at the national level that reinforced more local efforts, including:

- Food-labelling laws being changed so that salt and fat content was specified, making it easier to find and select low-salt and low-fat options
- Adopting school lunch policies that mandated healthier menus
- Dairy subsidies being dropped so that butter did not have a price advantage over low-fat alternatives
- Bread companies being lobbied to reduce salt and butter in their recipes, and sausage companies learning that it was possible to make and market a low-cholesterol product
- The Sports Act being passed in 1980, obliging the national and local governments to provide physical activity facilities

Case Analysis

The research questions laid out in chapter 4 shape the case analysis in this section. In particular, it is important to consider how the context and content of prevention educators in North Karelia compare with, and offer a perspective on, the CPE program in British Columbia.

Parallels with British Columbia and the CPE Program

GEOGRAPHICAL SETTING

The correct level of geographical comparison with British Columbia would have to be the entire country of Finland rather than the region of North Karelia. Finland and British Columbia have similar populations (~4 to 5 million), although British Columbia occupies about three times the land mass. Thus, North Karelia, one of 20 regions in Finland, can be legitimately equated with one of the areas assigned to CPEs in the province of British Columbia. The population of North Karelia would be roughly equivalent to the *average* "catchment" of a CPE in the province of British Columbia. This means that it is theoretically appropriate to draw comparisons between the prevention work of the North Karelia Project and that being pursued by a CPE in any one area of British Columbia.

North Karelia is mainly characterized by small villages, and this may make the project in that province more applicable to rural and remote areas of British Columbia rather than to the more urban regions. Even the capital city, Joensuu, is a relatively small centre, with a population of approximately 73,000. In the 1970s, the chief occupations in North Karelia were farming and forestry, which again is reminiscent of areas of British Columbia beyond the major cities.

FOCUS AND APPROACH

There has been a parallel interest in British Columbia and North Karelia (and Finland as a whole) in the common risk factors for chronic disease. Similarities in progress on such risk factors can also be identified, such as dropping rates of tobacco use. Another risk factor overlap has emerged as leaders in both Finland and British Columbia increasingly shift their focus to the behavioural factor of physical inactivity and the biological factor of overweight/obesity and its co-morbidities.

It is intriguing that the CPE program in British Columbia and the North Karelia Project are both strongly influenced by various theoretical frameworks. One of the mottos of the leaders in North Karelia has been: "nothing is as practical as a good theory." An example of a theory that shaped their practice is known as the "diffusion of innovations," a framework that was formalized by Rogers in a seminal book in 1962. Several elements enter into an understanding of the diffusion perspective: the innovation itself, the types of communication channels involved with getting news out about the innovation, the rate of adoption, and the social system that provides the context for individual and group acceptance of innovations. This complex of elements was implicated in developments in North Karelia on both a small scale (e.g., the work of lay opinion leaders) and a large scale (e.g., the spread of the project vision throughout Finland). The latter experience, where programs and approaches being piloted in North Karelia were adapted and adopted in other parts of the country, offers another alignment with the B.C. situation. Thus, aspects of the CPE program that first began in the southern interior of British Columbia are now part of the network established throughout the province.

TEAM CHARACTERISTICS

The high-level alignment of key North Karelia Project staff members with the features of a CPE was already introduced in chapter 4: they were professionals coordinating prevention efforts for a defined population in a manner marked by a generalist focus and community engagement. Beyond these basic facts, there are further similarities, as well as differences, between project workers in North Karelia and CPEs in British Columbia. First, the community-based workers in North Karelia were drawn from professions similar to those found on the résumés of CPEs, especially nurses and nutritionists. Another important similarity is that the initiators of the project in North Karelia were local, and thus very familiar with the issues, context, and stakeholders. Furthermore, some of the project leaders were involved over a number of years, again building the "local knowledge" foundation for ensuing prevention efforts. For example, the medical officer position in North Karelia was occupied by the same person from 1978 to 1997. One advantage of the stability in personnel in the North Karelia Project was the ability to identify and recruit the most influential local opinion leaders and lay workers. This is reminiscent of the desire in the British Columbia Cancer Agency to hire CPEs with existing professional and/ or personal linkages to the region where they will be serving.

Contrasts with British Columbia and the CPE Program

POLITICAL SETTING
Health services are mostly organized on a regional basis in British Columbia, with leadership specific to each of five regional health authorities, but the historic pattern of governance in Finland exists on two levels: the state as a whole and the municipality. The entire land area of Finland is currently divided into 342 municipalities. The point and practice of municipal organization historically had a socioeconomic foundation: the boundaries were defined by how far one could travel by horse in one day, from home to the main village centre and back again by nightfall. This deeply rooted tradition of socioeconomic organization persists today, albeit with the horse replaced by the automobile, allowing for centuries-old municipalities to sometimes be amalgamated into larger units for more efficient operation in the contemporary world.

Contrary to how cities and towns are positioned in the Canadian political landscape (i.e., overshadowed by the authority vested in provincial and territorial governments), municipalities in Finland are where the formal and real power lies for all decisions located below the national level, including those related to health services. The Regional Council of North Karelia, for instance, is a body with only limited duties authorized by a federation of the 14 municipalities of North Karelia; it appears to be occupied mostly with economic matters, higher education, and partnerships with the European Union, but not with health care.

The involvement of so many Finnish political units with health care decisions offers both challenges and opportunities when compared with the regional organization in British Columbia. According to Professor Vartiainen, it is difficult for the smaller municipalities to afford and operate tertiary-level services such as a hospital. However, targeted, community-level prevention programs may be customized and rolled out more effectively in the context of local government.

SPECIFIC POPULATIONS

British Columbia has some unique challenges to contend with in terms of isolated First Nations (Aboriginal) communities. Furthermore, the health care needs of Aboriginal peoples living on reserves (hereditary land tracts with generally collective ownership of title) are jurisdictionally the responsibility of the federal government, which can lead to some complications related to "turf issues." Modern-day Finland and Canada (including British Columbia) both have to address cultural competency in health care and other social arenas, especially in the context of immigrant populations. The type and prevalence of ethnocultural groups differ in the two settings. Compared to most other upper-income countries, the inflow of foreign citizens, immigrants, and refugees into Finland in modern times started relatively late, in the early 1990s; this means that up until recently the country has been ethnically homogeneous, lessening the pressure to respond to cross-cultural health care needs.

FOCUS AND APPROACH

The most obvious contrast with the *cancer* focus of CPEs in British Columbia is the consistent targeting of *cardiovascular disease* risk factors in the North Karelia Project. Two realities mitigate this divergence somewhat. First, there has been evidence of a collateral benefit in terms of cancer incidence in North Karelia. The second point is closely connected to the first: It involves the fact that the cardiovascular risk factors of interest in North Karelia, namely, unhealthy diets and tobacco use, are also implicated in the development of many cancers. Thus, the work of the North Karelia Project and the activities of CPEs are not as far apart as may first appear.

Compared to the North Karelia Project, a CPE has a mandate larger than primary prevention, specifically including activities related to classic secondary prevention efforts related to cancer screening. As for the work in North Karelia, there appeared to be more attention paid to risk factor screening and medical interventions based in the primary care arena.

Another distinction is the time and place of the North Karelia Project, specifically as it relates to the phenomenon of globalization. It was relatively easy 30 years ago to contact and influence the main food suppliers in an area such as North Karelia, but it is much more difficult to accomplish this in the highly interconnected world of today, where whole and processed food is transported hundreds and even thousands of miles to reach markets in the various parts of a province like British Columbia. This suggests that the process of influencing the food environment will require efforts beyond the community, and involve players beyond community-based prevention educators.

In both North Karelia and British Columbia, the emphasis has been more "bottom up" rather than "top down" in terms of program development and adoption. There has been a strong commitment to work with influential contacts in community organizations, as well as networking across a range of social platforms for change (schools, businesses, local government, etc.). However, the North Karelia Project appears to have gone even further, with more intentional and systematic recruiting of lay workers and opinion leaders to help diffuse the prevention message throughout the region. Versions of this model may occur informally when a particular CPE in British Columbia is focused on a specific ethnocultural group.

TEAM CHARACTERISTICS
While both the North Karelia team and the CPE program represent a professional effort that is ultimately operated by government funding and under a government umbrella, a contrast may be drawn between them. Because of the intermediary role of a quasi-government group (the British Columbia Cancer Agency) in recruiting and supervision, and because CPEs are drawn from many walks of life and are often contracted rather than hired as full-time employees, it may be that the CPE approach is not recognized by clients and potential partners as an official or authorized extension of government health work. Although it is a subtle distinction, this may account for the fact that the North Karelia Project was able to generate more involvement with (and reorientation of) primary care resources. Indeed, this marshalling of health care services, including clinical prevention measures for high-risk individuals,

is an important difference between the work in North Karelia and the work in British Columbia.

On the other hand, it should be acknowledged that there are trade-offs between the influence at the disposal of government officers and the scepticism and resistance that such individuals may encounter. It is true that the more collaborative or negotiation-based approach required of an "unofficial" worker (such as a CPE) is more time-consuming and sometimes frustrating, but the ultimate fruit in terms of grassroots ownership may be more substantial and sustained. In fact, Dr Puska underlined strongly that the staff (and program) of the North Karelia Project enjoyed a unique dual character, both official/governmental and more community-connected and non-governmental. They alternated between each mode as required, for example, being able to partner with industry in a way that would be more problematic for representatives of a pure government program. Indeed, the North Karelia Project was able to set up a foundation to facilitate private fundraising.

Insights for CPE (and Similar) Programs

There are several clear lessons that may be drawn from North Karelia for a CPE program as it currently operates in British Columbia, and for similar strategies that may be considered for implementation in other jurisdictions.

First, the value of a number of characteristic elements of the CPE program is reinforced by the example of North Karelia, including:

- Local translation of health promotion knowledge to benefit one or more defined populations
- Collaboration with a variety of health-related organizations
- Being strongly rooted in theory, comprising health promotion in general and then more specific concepts and applications
- Generally, a commitment to work in a "bottom up" rather than a "top down" manner, fostering as much community engagement as possible

In sum, North Karelia offers solid encouragement for the paradigm that is being pursued in British Columbia. The Finnish program stands as an example of what a grassroots community-oriented primary prevention program with sustained funding over more than 30 years can accomplish.

Second, it seems that deploying a team (rather than a solo worker) to work in each area has advantages both in terms of multiple skill sets being brought together and in the potential for joint strategizing. The CPE role may sometimes feel lonely, especially in more remote parts of British Columbia. Quantitatively, there is also the basic issue of staff-to-population ratio. This is much less favourable in British Columbia, possibly intensifying a sense of being overwhelmed and needing to manage a serious time deficit. While acknowledging that there usually will be substantial budgetary implications attached to a higher staff-to-population ratio, significantly expanding the number of CPEs in British Columbia would increase the opportunity for teamwork, improve the quality of prevention coordination, possibly enhance a sense of professional satisfaction, and ultimately, based on the evidence, lead to a more effective prevention program.

Third, investing in a (demonstrably successful) pilot project and then transferring the momentum and lessons to other geographical areas has worked well in British Columbia and Finland. The North Karelia Project likely enhanced the diffusion process with its commitment to generating high-quality data on processes and (especially) health outcomes. Connected to this pattern was the fostering among practitioners of close working relationships with scientists in North Karelia, including both epidemiologists and intervention designers/evaluators.

Fourth, the North Karelia Project generally represented a more substantial form of integration of health care for the purpose of prevention than typically has been possible in a jurisdiction such as British Columbia. Ultimately, one must work within one's contexts and constraints. British Columbia in the 2000s is different than Finland in the 1970s; in particular, there are unique forms of "resistance" to health care integration in the contemporary Canadian setting. Nonetheless, the desire to see more levels of partnership, especially with primary care resources geared to prevention, should continue to motivate improvements in the CPE model.

Fifth, all strategies to reduce risk exposure and consequent disease must be marshalled in the battle against the burden of chronic conditions. Professor Vartiainen noted that two different movements in public health often seem to exist in isolation from one another, one focusing on traditional risk factor reduction and disease control, and the other on health promotion and/or social determinants. Vartiainen maintained that a big part of the success of the North Karelia Project involved not opposing these two domains but instead integrating them. In short, combining medical and public health efforts with strategies focused on changing social determinants is vital to the sort of progress on chronic disease reduction that is required in every jurisdiction.

Although it is fair to say that the full expression of the social determinants perspective in Finland has happened more recently in the so-called "Health in All Policies" initiative, the North Karelia Project generated broader involvement among sectors outside of health services from the start. The application to a CPE-type program may be summed up as follows: to redouble efforts in both clinical and community-level prevention while attempting to pursue new insights and initiatives related to social determinants.

Finally, it is apparent that long-term commitment to a region is vital. Change agency, whether directed at individuals, communities, or the wider society, requires trust-building and other forms of careful, patient investment over time. Dr Puska's "mantra" for success in a comprehensive, community-based effort was: do the right things, and do enough of them. To this may be added the importance of a "long obedience in the same direction" (to paraphrase Nietzsche). Dr Puska reminisced that the person who recruited him maintained that "hiring you was the best decision, not because you were good, but because you were young!" The implication was that he and the other leaders would have staying power. It is remarkable that 40 years later Drs. Vartiainen and Puska occupy adjoining offices at the same institute in Helsinki, and that they continue to eloquently transmit the North Karelia story.

Conclusion

More than 35 years of results and experiences of the North Karelia Project show that a determined and well-conceived set of interventions can have a tremendous impact on health-related lifestyles and on population risk factor levels, and that such a development can lead to reduced disease rates and improved population health. The dramatic success, so dependent on the dedication and skills of staff people focused on a needy and motivated population, helps to explain why a program in a relatively small and remote Finnish province has been so influential in that country and eventually around the world. The lessons have been considered and applied in other settings, from Iran to India, from Scotland to Sweden. This has even been happening since the 1990s in the neighbouring Karelian region of the Russian Federation, creating a health partnership "bridge" that should go a long way to healing a political divide instigated by decades-old conflicts.

Adaptation to nearby Nordic settings could be somewhat easier than translating the North Karelian principles to jurisdictions such as China, Chile, or even British Columbia, but ultimately the vital effort to improve chronic disease prevention in both higher-income and lower- and middle-income parts of the world needs to draw on insights wherever they may be found.

Sources and Further Reading

North Karelia Project

Hendley J, Gorman RM. Miracle up north. *Eating Well* online newsletter. Available at http://www.eatingwell.com/nutrition_health/nutrition_news_information/miracle_up_north (accessed 8 January 2012).

Luostarinen T, Hakulinen T, Pukkala E. Cancer risk following a community-based programme to prevent cardiovascular diseases. Int J Epidemiol. 1995;24(6):1094–9. http://dx.doi.org/10.1093/ije/24.6.1094. Medline:8824849

McAlister A, Puska P, Salonen JT, et al. Theory and action for health promotion illustrations from the North Karelia Project. Am J Public Health. 1982;72(1):43–50. http://dx.doi.org/10.2105/AJPH.72.1.43. Medline:7053618

Papadakis S, Moroz I. Population-level interventions for coronary heart disease prevention: what have we learned since the North Karelia project? Curr Opin Cardiol. 2008;23(5):452–61. http://dx.doi.org/10.1097/HCO.0b013e32830c217e. Medline:18670256

Puska P. The North Karelia Project: 30 years successfully preventing chronic diseases. Diabetes Voice. 2008;53:26–9.

Puska P, Vartiainen E, Laatikainen T, et al. *The North Karelia Project: From North Karelia to National Action.* Helsinki: Helsinki University Printing House; 2009.

Vartiainen E, Laatikainen T, Peltonen M, et al. Thirty-five-year trends in cardiovascular risk factors in Finland. Int J Epidemiol. 2010;39(2):504–18. http://dx.doi.org/10.1093/ije/dyp330. Medline:19959603

Other Topics

Kreindler SA. Lifting the burden of chronic disease: what has worked? what hasn't? what's next? Healthc Q. 2009;12(2):30–40. Medline:19369809

Krueger H, Williams D, Kaminsky B, et al. *The Health Impact of Smoking and Obesity and What to Do about It.* Toronto: University of Toronto Press; 2007.

Multiple Risk Factor Intervention Trial Research Group. Multiple risk factor intervention trial. Risk factor changes and mortality results. JAMA. 1982;248(12):1465–77. http://dx.doi.org/10.1001/jama.1982.03330120023025. Medline:7050440

Puska P, Ståhl T. Health in all policies-the Finnish initiative: background, principles, and current issues. [Epub ahead of print]. Annu Rev Public Health. 2010;31(1):315–28, 3, 328. http://dx.doi.org/10.1146/annurev.publhealth.012809.103658. Medline:20070201

Romon M, Lommez A, Tafflet M, et al. Downward trends in the prevalence of childhood overweight in the setting of 12-year school- and community-based programmes. Public Health Nutr. 2009;12(10):1735–42. http://dx.doi.org/10.1017/S1368980008004278. Medline:19102807

Saaristo T, Etu-Seppala L. Prevention of diabetes and its complications: key goals in Finland. Diabetes Voice. 2006;51:13–7.

Shea S, Basch CE. A review of five major community-based cardiovascular disease prevention programs. Part II: Intervention strategies, evaluation methods, and results. Am J Health Promot. 1990;4(4):279–87. http://dx.doi.org/10.4278/0890-1171-4.4.279. Medline:10106505

Vlasoff T, Laatikainen T, Korpelainen V, et al. Ten year trends in chronic disease risk factors in the Republic of Karelia, Russia. Eur J Public Health. 2008;18(6):666–73. http://dx.doi.org/10.1093/eurpub/ckn063. Medline:18628317

6 Northern Ireland: Health Promotion Officers

Sean was at the end of a long day: exhausted, yes, but in a good way. He had spent the last few hours in Carnmoney, a town of fewer than 3,000 people on the outskirts of Belfast, Northern Ireland's largest city. There, in a shopping mall parking lot, he had met one-on-one with a large number of local citizens in Action Cancer's "Big Bus." Sean had provided brief personalized health checks for a variety of chronic disease and cancer-specific risk factors. It was busier than they had expected, no doubt as a result of a story that had run on the local news the night before promoting the mobile services available through the Big Bus. One particular case stuck in his mind as he finished packing up with the other members of his team. It had been a mid-day meeting with a man in his early thirties. The evidence of skin damage from sun exposure was apparent right away. Although this was a common occurrence, it was still shocking in someone so young. Due to the fair skin and other genetic predispositions among individuals of Irish descent, skin cancer is a constant concern. As he passed along this information, Sean learned that the man's father had died of melanoma just a year before. Sean promised himself that he would add extra emphasis to his classroom visit in the following week, where one of the topics was the correct application of sunscreens. In the meantime, noting that the man was also a smoker, Sean discussed the risks of continuing to smoke and made sure he also took along a readiness-to-quit brochure. Now it was time to take the Big Bus back to home base and get ready for another town, another parking lot, and another lineup of clients on the following day.

This case study will reflect on the work of Action Cancer in Northern Ireland, and particularly its team of health promotion officers. Emily

Magrath, the current manager of health promotion, was a valuable informant regarding the work of the team and other aspects of Action Cancer. This organization, which has established itself as a leader in cancer detection and prevention through a variety of innovative programs, is unique in the programs analysed in this book because it operates as a private charity. In fact, it is the largest (by income) cancer-related charity in Northern Ireland. Despite its non-governmental status, Action Cancer (and particularly its health promotion department) shares a number of characteristics with the CPE program in British Columbia and other similar regionalized prevention programs.

Development of Action Cancer

Action Cancer was established in 1973 by Dr George Edelstyn. The charity actually initiated breast and cervical screening programs in Northern Ireland in 1978, a full 10 years before the National Health Service (NHS) introduced similar programs. To date, approximately 100,000 women have used these services at Action Cancer House in Belfast. In general, its early detection clinics and mobile screening units (see below) have aimed to promote cancer-avoiding behaviours and a personal commitment to screening, particularly in rural areas and socially deprived, inner-city communities.

The organization continues to pursue its founder's vision of freeing the people of Northern Ireland from the burden of cancer. Among its many innovations is a men's health program, started in 1997, that offers an evening clinic for men concerned about prostate or testicular cancer. Augmenting efforts among this sometimes neglected demographic group, an annual men's campaign is undertaken to raise awareness about male-specific cancers and to encourage men to seek help if they have a concern.

Although not a direct part of the NHS, Action Cancer, along with other cancer charities in the Northern Ireland Cancer Network, are generally trusted partners in the fight against cancer. For instance, in 1998, Action Cancer established a cancer information service situated adjacent to Belfast City Hospital, the regional cancer centre. Staffed by cancer information specialists and volunteers, the service provided information on all aspects of cancer, early detection and screening programs, counselling, and practical help available to cancer patients and their families.

The acknowledgment of the voluntary sector and its integration with government cancer services in Northern Ireland has varied. Certainly,

Table 6.1   Action Cancer Funding and Expenditures, 2008/2009

Funding			Expenditures		
	%	£		%	£
Shops	25	886,784	Health Promotion and Prevention	15	530,011
Community Fundraising	15	532,070	Breast Screening Service	19	671,347
Special Events	15	532,070	Regional, Development, and Big Bus	18	636,013
Individual Donations and Legacies	21	744,899	Cancer Support and Information	11	388,675
Corporate Fundraising	12	425,656	Campaigns and Fundraising	13	459,343
Trusts and Foundations	4	141,885	Trading Costs	11	388,675
Investments, Marketing and Other Income	8	283,771	Cancer Research	8	282,672
			Governance	4	141,336
Total	100	3,547,136	Total	99	3,533,406

Note: Component amounts calculated by applying percentage to totals, and are therefore approximate. Percentages may not total 100 because of rounding.

Source: Action Cancer, *Annual Review 2008/2009*

from the perspective of Action Cancer, there has been an effort to complement government services rather than duplicate them. For instance, Emily Magrath noted that once the NHS breast cancer screening service was established for women aged 50–69, Action Cancer concentrated on providing mammography for women aged 40–49 and 70-plus.

As shown in Table 6.1, funding for the charity comes from a variety of sources, including individual donations, corporate and community sources, special events, trusts and foundations, and investments and marketing. Remarkably, there is little or no public funding for the operation of Action Cancer, apart from modest grants for specific projects.

The funds received are instrumental in supporting various programs. Services are sometimes tailored to gender or age groups, and are often delivered in a regionalized and/or mobile manner. In addition to client and population-wide activities, allocations are made to support research at local universities; these grants are used to study both prevention and treatment, with a recent focus on researching the social impact of cancer on family members and communities.

Ultimately, the purpose of Action Cancer has become distilled into four objectives:

1. Early detection of cancer
2. Support services for cancer patients and those close to them
3. Health promotion services for men, women, and children
4. Funding for local cancer research

Key Programs and Activities

Action Cancer makes use of broad media and marketing efforts, sometimes involving celebrity spokespersons; they have evidence to back up this strategic commitment of resources. For instance, an older study of their cancer information telephone line showed that almost 18% of the annual inquiries related to the discovery of breast changes were reported during October, which was Breast Cancer Awareness month. During that period, Action Cancer's breast awareness campaign was extensive, involving billboard advertising, newspaper articles, and television and radio spots. Similarly, Action Cancer's Safe Sun campaign led to significant referrals. The pigmented lesion clinics, promoted and supported by Action Cancer as part of that campaign, resulted in the detection of nine skin cancers, including two melanomas, and led to surgical treatment in over 50% of all specialist referrals generated through general practitioner consultations.

In addition to high-profile media campaigns, Action Cancer is probably best known for the tangible resource known as the Big Bus. With sponsorship from the firm SuperValu, the Big Bus was designed by Action Cancer staff, constructed, and then launched in August 2006. Originally conceived as a re-purposed double-decker bus, the project eventually ended up adapting a 14-metre trailer pulled by a Volvo tractor. The trailer has extendable pods to increase the service area inside. Although it ultimately did not involve a bus, the original name stuck.

Travelling to 200 communities in Northern Ireland each year, the Big Bus serves as a self-contained, multipurpose mobile unit, capable of delivering services that span the spectrum of cancer prevention, as well as offering some aspects of cancer care. It represents an expansion of a previous mobile service that focused on breast and cervical screening and breast cancer awareness education. Over the years, a reported 55,000 people have used the mobile early detection services of Action Cancer. This effort has been enhanced recently through the purchase of new mammography units that use a lower radiation dose and provide better imaging of the dense breast tissue that is common in younger women. The focus on breast cancer screening is understandable. Over 1,000 women in Northern Ireland are diagnosed with breast cancer each year, and around 300 die annually from the disease. Action Cancer invests almost 20% of its budget in this aspect of the screening program, with a good "return" on this commitment of resources; the program is responsible for the detection of about 5% of all breast cancers diagnosed in Northern Ireland.

Programs offered by Action Cancer, and uptake by cancer patients and their families, have gradually expanded. For example, over 10,000 clients have accessed counselling care services to date. In addition to early detection and support services, health promotion activity is undertaken with men and women in the workplace and in community groups, and with children and adolescents in school settings. Action Cancer's school-based promotion programs have been in place, in one form or another, since 1996. Initially using an interactive "magic" show to highlight the importance of healthy eating, exercise, and safe sun practices with primary school students, the program has evolved and expanded to secondary schools and colleges. Health Action was launched in 2009 for young people aged 11 to 18 (with special funding from the independent retail chain Centra). The four hour-long sessions typical of the program are designed to cover:

• Tobacco and alcohol use
• Being body aware and building self-esteem
• Health eating and exercise
• Cardiobox or dancercise demonstrations (and participation)

The £500,000 in funding contributed by Centra over 6 years led to a temporary expansion of the health promotion team. This increase in staffing has been important, allowing for outreach to about 30,000 young people annually since 2003. While many aspects of Action Cancer are very visible in Northern Ireland society, arguably its less visible "backbone" is the team of regionally situated health promotion officers

(HPOs). As outlined further in the next section, they are essential to a variety of primary and secondary prevention programs that highlight lifestyle factors and raise awareness about the symptoms of cancer and the importance of early detection.

Regional Health Promotion Team

Action Cancer's regional health promotion team currently has six staff members and a manager; all are professionals with postsecondary degrees. The consistent standard of entry for this sort of work in Northern Ireland is a diploma in health promotion. A solid educational foundation is important, although in most cases extensive on-the-job training is also required to master the large number of services that each HPO is expected to provide. These include school talks aimed at various age groups, sessions for community groups, programs in workplaces, smoking cessation counselling, and health checks (described below). Ms Magrath noted that it typically takes a year for an HPO to be fully equipped for his or her role. In the end, each HPO is prepared to offer the extensive range of services, including all types of health messages. The only break they get is from operating the puppet used in preschool and elementary school talks known as Wally & Wise: for those events a sessional contract is arranged with a professional puppeteer!

The health promotion program has operated out of four different offices spread around Northern Ireland; the locations are Belfast, Londonderry, Newry, and Magherafelt (see Figure 6.1). Staff turnover and the requirements of team-building have led to the majority of officers currently residing in or near Belfast, but there is still a commitment to regional work with an assigned population. It is also true that a large proportion of the province's population lives in the east near Belfast. The city is the home of the organization's headquarters, Action Cancer House, where many members of the health promotion team are based, including the program manager.

Two priorities permeate every program implemented by these cancer workers: primary prevention, aimed at behavioural changes that can help to prevent over 50% of cancers, and early detection and diagnosis (with the goal of successful treatment and longer survival).

Health education is clearly at the heart of the role played by HPOs. The lifestyle targets include classic risk factors such as smoking, diet, exercise, alcohol, stress, and ultraviolet radiation exposure. The parallel communication agenda involves raising awareness of common

Figures 6.1. Map of Northern Ireland.

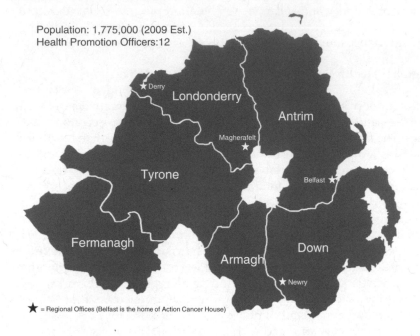

Population: 1,775,000 (2009 Est.)
Health Promotion Officers:12

★ = Regional Offices (Belfast is the home of Action Cancer House)

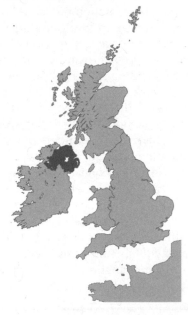

symptoms of specific cancers, sometimes in the context of motivating people to take advantage of early detection services. HPOs deliver these two sets of messages in a variety of settings, from schools to workplaces to adult community groups. A number of educational formats are employed, from public sessions on healthy living or cancer awareness to nutrition classes known as "Cook-It." The latter sessions provide information about healthy eating while cooking recommended recipes as a group. With a focus on inexpensive and practical menus, Cook-It covers breakfast, lunch, and dinner; it promotes nutritious but palatable choices such as whole-wheat pancakes, sweet and sour stir-fry, and root vegetable korma.

In recent years, Action Cancer introduced "MOT" health checks, offered either at fixed clinics or as part of a visit to the Big Bus. MOT, a term originally coined by the Ministry of Transport, denotes the yearly checks of roadworthiness required for vehicles over 3 years old. Applied as a metaphor to the health arena, it is now used to refer to an annual check of health status made available to both men and women over 16 years of age. During an informal (but still confidential) 15-minute session, individuals are presented with a menu of testing options, including:

- *Cholesterol.* A small sample from a finger prick allows for a full analysis of serum fats (cholesterol and triglycerides).
- *Blood pressure and pulse rate.* Of course, high blood pressure has implications beyond cancer, specifically in the area of cardiovascular disease.
- *Body-mass index.* Height and weight measurements allow BMI to be calculated.
- *Body composition analysis.* Measures body fat percentage through the use of electrical signals.
- *Facial skin scanner analysis.* A rapid measurement of skin condition, the scanner is able to show damage that has occurred due to UV exposure, which may be a precursor of skin cancer.
- *Lung capacity.* The Pulmolife machine checks lung function, offering an indication the lung's "physiologic age."

Following analysis, HPOs take the opportunity to discuss the results, integrating additional health messaging as appropriate. Depending on the checklist that clients take away, they may be encouraged to follow up with their general practitioners.

Case Analysis

Comparisons with British Columbia and the CPE Program

GEOGRAPHICAL COVERAGE

Northern Ireland covers a land area of approximately 14,000 km^2, less than one seventh that of British Columbia; it has a population of 1.8 million, fewer than half of the B.C. population and slightly fewer than the number of people in the Metro Vancouver area of British Columbia. The current complement of six HPOs operating in Northern Ireland represents an approximate ratio of 1:300,000 citizens, or a similar "order of magnitude" as the CPE program in British Columbia.

The regionalization is less structured in Northern Ireland, as the small sub-teams of HPOs operate out of only four centres. This creates the advantage of more regular, active teamwork, in contrast with the more solo functioning of the CPEs. On the other hand, target populations are less narrowly defined in Northern Ireland.

The program delivery offered by HPOs is often directly connected with the mobile resource of the Big Bus, possibly creating a more fluid sense of geographical boundaries for each HPO's assignment. This sense of being "assigned" to the whole country rather than a specific region would be reinforced by the fact that travel distances in Northern Ireland are much less than in British Columbia.

Northern Ireland represents a much more ethnically uniform population base than British Columbia. Over 99% of the citizens of Northern Ireland are Caucasian. In contrast, the large, sometimes concentrated minority groups in British Columbia require a greater awareness of cultural competency issues, which has sometimes led to the recruiting of culture-specific CPEs.

FOCUS AND APPROACH

The Action Cancer charity operates across a broad platform, with the health promotion team representing one focal point within the continuum of cancer care. This is similar to the relationship between CPEs and the British Columbia Cancer Agency (BCCA). The BCCA is responsible for a wide range of services, including very advanced and even experimental treatments. Another interesting parallel is that the BCCA also operates a mobile screening service (specifically, mammography for woman aged 40–79), although using smaller vehicles that cannot accommodate the range of services provided on the Big Bus.

Both the CPE program and Action Cancer HPOs focus on cancer primary prevention through changing health behaviours and thereby modifying risk factor prevalence; of course, the risk factors of interest are relevant to a variety of chronic diseases. Again, both CPEs and HPOs are involved with secondary prevention efforts, specifically screening and early detection of cancer. The balance between these two service arenas differs between the two jurisdictions. While early detection represents an equal, if not dominant, focus for HPOs in Northern Ireland, it generally represents a much smaller part of the CPE agenda. It is true that a shift may be occurring in this regard, with a number of CPEs beginning to spend more time promoting screening services.

A more subtle distinction may be seen in the execution of the primary prevention mandate. While both CPEs and HPOs may be characterized as generalists in their perspectives and activities, the workers in Northern Ireland are better defined as program deliverers. In fact, they are involved in what may be fairly described as clinical services, such as face-to-face health checks, counselling, etc. HPOs concentrate on assessing and/or informing individuals or perhaps small groups; the success of their approach may be measured in terms of convincing clients to make better choices about their health. In contrast, CPEs typically work more on the community level, influencing other leaders to change the environment and remove any obstacles standing in the way of making healthy choices. In summary, the Action Cancer model is not based so much on the "classical" definition of health promotion, since the work of the HPOs tends towards an individualistic, educational approach as opposed to a broader community engagement. The approach of the CPEs, in contrast, reflects the premise: "knowing better does not automatically lead to doing better."

PRIVATE CHARITY VERSUS GOVERNMENT

There is irony in the distinction just described between classic health promotion focusing on community change and health education focusing on individual change. One would expect more attention to the former within the Action Cancer world, since it is a charity. Organizations such as Action Cancer, which do not rely at all on government funding, typically have more freedom to collaborate on the advocacy activities that often flow from (and lead to) community engagement. It is true, as one might expect, that direct advocacy is not on the agenda of quasi-governmental CPEs either; nonetheless, they are generally *more* involved with community development efforts than are the HPOs in Northern Ireland.

The BCCA's status as a quasi-governmental body has both advantages and limitations when compared to the full charity status of Action Cancer. For instance, there is a greater possibility of integrating primary and secondary prevention efforts with other aspects of cancer care and treatment. As well, the cancer agency in British Columbia does not have to spend time and resources on fundraising. Positioning the efforts of Action Cancer for maximum public relations impact is a constant concern, and could even affect program priorities. This reality may have led to the emphasis on clinical services in the Action Cancer portfolio; success stories involving individuals generally "play" more strongly in the media than population-wide changes.

On the other hand, Action Cancer and similar bodies in British Columbia (e.g., the Canadian Cancer Society) do have the ability and know-how to raise substantial funds to apply to the fight against cancer; they also have the freedom to enter into arrangements with corporate sponsors that are not appropriate for government agencies. At the heart of this strategy lies a strong communications department that creates sponsorships and designs advertising campaigns. Most important of all, independently funded organizations such as Action Cancer can choose to make primary prevention a true priority, while it sometimes seems to exist as a "poor cousin" within government health departments.

Finally, there are complex issues around how a government officer is perceived as compared with a private agent. Other non-governmental organizations may feel more comfortable working with staff from a similar type of group. However, as discussed in the chapter on the North Karelia Project, it is possible for government-funded agents to operate in a "non-official" manner; this flexible profile is probably exploited in a similar way by CPEs in British Columbia.

Insights for the CPE (and Similar) Programs

The Action Cancer model of HPOs reinforces the value of similar elements from the CPE program, namely:

- A regionalized approach with a more-or-less defined population target for each leader
- Focusing on a range of risk factors that are relevant across gender and age groups, including both cancer-specific factors and those

that are common to many chronic diseases; there is thus a celebration of the "generalist" role in both Action Cancer and the CPE program (as opposed to workers who specialize in, for instance, smoking cessation)

- Recognizing the dual importance of primary prevention and secondary prevention (as represented by screening and early detection), although Action Cancer's commitment to practical integration of these arenas has gone further

On the latter point, it may be strategic to incorporate one or more expanded mobile units into the work of a CPE-like program. Of course, the capital and operating budget for such a resource is always an issue. It is not clear that private sponsorship (and branding) would ever be as appropriate for government agencies as it is for the voluntary sector. If the funding stream could be established in an acceptable way, mobile services could be very attractive in any jurisdiction with large rural regions. In addition to increasing access to services, they are a high-profile tool with many opportunities for publicity; media reports and advertising could have collateral benefit in terms of drawing attention to other health promotion efforts.

A related strategic question is whether it would ever be feasible to truly bring together the more educational and clinical services favoured by the Action Cancer program and the community engagement and development functions that are part of the classic health promotion focus on social determinants. Aspects of the CPE program currently exist behind the scenes, specifically the collaborative work with community groups and organizations. Of course, the community health education work of CPEs does pull them into the public eye; however, an even stronger presence among the general public through one-to-one services may be valuable to the overall prevention agenda. The obvious barriers to such a development include the limitations of their part-time status and the very large regions that must be covered by the CPEs in British Columbia.

Conclusion

Publicity and public relations are complicated categories to interpret in the context of prevention programs. They consume a lot of time, creative energy, and expense. On the other hand, properly leveraged, publicity can augment the effectiveness of other interventions by encouraging awareness, uptake, adherence, etc. As well, in the context of a private charity, there is freedom to enter into endorsement and sponsorship arrangements that can be very helpful for fundraising, as well as for getting the message out. An example of Action Cancer using both strategies is the "smoker's face" campaign, which was sponsored by Gordons Chemists. It started with a recent photograph of popular television presenter and former Miss Northern Ireland, Zoe Salmon; the image was then digitally modified to look as though she had been smoking since the age of 15. The photo was meant to appeal to concerns shared by some young people about physical appearance. It is unclear whether the CPE program or the British Columbia Cancer Agency as a whole would ever be able to match the publicity mechanisms available to an organization such as Action Cancer. In some sense, this book, with its full description of the CPE program, is an attempt to redress the publicity gap by getting the story out to those who will be inspired to "go and do likewise."

Sources and Further Reading

Action Cancer. *Reflections on the Past Year - Annual Review 2009/10*. 2010. Available at http://www.actioncancer.org/ActionCancerSite/files/04/04b5836a-5e0e-4c56-9403-7a37822c5970.pdf (accessed July 2011).

Action Cancer. *A Continuing Future - Strategic Plan 2010–2013*. 2010. Available at http://www.actioncancer.org/ActionCancerSite/files/8c/8ce76ca8-999e-4a67-a171-548fa57902a5.PDF (accessed July 2011).

Heenan D. A partnership approach to health promotion: a case study from Northern Ireland. Health Promot Int. 2004;19(1):105–13. http://dx.doi.org/10.1093/heapro/dah111. Medline:14976178

Manning DL, Quigley P. Understanding the needs of people using a cancer information service in Northern Ireland. Eur J Cancer Care (Engl). 2002;11(2):139–42. http://dx.doi.org/10.1046/j.1365-2354.2002.00299.x. Medline:12099950

Owen T, Fitzpatrick D, Dolan O, et al. Knowledge, attitudes and behaviour in the sun: the barriers to behavioural change in Northern Ireland. Ulster Med J. 2004;73(2):96–104. Medline:15651769

Regional Cancer Framework. A Cancer Control Programme for Northern Ireland. Available at http://www.dhsspsni.gov.uk/eeu_cancer_control_programme_eqia.pdf (accessed 23 January 2010).

7 Kentucky: Cooperative Extension Agents and Cancer Control Specialists

In the words of University of Kentucky President Lee T. Todd Jr, "Extension agents throughout the state are in daily contact with individuals and families. They are our best ambassadors and have a forum to mobilize communities to improve their health." In a seminal speech, he likens the health education workers to a business sales force. As a former corporate executive, Todd led teams of sales people. In his experience then, the relevant personnel were not always located in all the areas where they are needed; as a happy contrast, he inherited "sales offices" with health extension agents in all 120 counties of Kentucky. He sees them as trusted ambassadors who can effectively carry health messages as the "product." Important traits of an effective salesperson include listening to the customers and providing feedback to the company's research department so that the product can be improved. Regionalized prevention leaders in Kentucky learn about the specific needs of community members and then relay the information back to university researchers so that programs may be developed or adapted accordingly. In this way, they act as a two-way communication channel, bridging the gap between academia and average Kentuckians.

The Health Education through Extension Leadership (HEEL) program based out of the University of Kentucky involves collaboration between the extension health specialists from the College of Nursing and cooperative extension agents who live and work in communities they serve. It represents a creative marriage of health care and agriculture, since extension agents have historically been strongly connected with farming and farm families. As a modern application of the Cooperative Extensive Service that goes back many decades throughout the United States, HEEL has a goal of decreasing or eliminating chronic disease through preventive health education and other interventions. The program relates strongly to other programs in Kentucky, further integrating the worlds of health care (e.g., the American Cancer Society) and agriculture (e.g., the 4-H movement). The Kentucky Cancer Program is one such partner organization; while displaying features that are unique in the U.S. setting, it does offer intriguing parallels with the CPE program in British Columbia.

This chapter will describe both HEEL and the KCP in more detail before building a case analysis of these two organizations and their regionalized approach to chronic disease prevention. The need for such initiatives in this particular state is very clear. The rates of cancer, diabetes, heart disease, and chronic obstructive pulmonary disease in Kentucky are among the highest in the United States. These indicators of poor health status, combined with the high rates of poverty and illiteracy, are sometimes collectively referred to as "the Kentucky uglies." Smoking, obesity, and high blood pressure, all behavioural risk factors for one or more the above-mentioned diseases, are also very prevalent in the state; according to 2006 data, Kentucky had the highest smoking rate in the United States at just over 28%, and was ranked seventh for obesity at 27.5%. There are several factors that contribute to the poor health status of Kentuckians, including the remote regions that are often marked by inadequate access to health care. In fact, approximately half of all Kentuckians live in rural areas, often isolated from any population centre; as a result, health care facilities are difficult to reach for many citizens. Lack of education, usually associated with lower health status, is also a substantial concern in Kentucky. While the rate of dropping out of high school has been gradually reduced, completion of postsecondary education in the state is lower than the national average; consistent with this statistic, Kentucky has the eighth-highest poverty rate in the United States.

HEEL Program

Historical Roots

The HEEL program was developed in 2001 as a result of a statewide health needs assessment. As noted above, the ultimate goal of the program is to reduce chronic disease rates by encouraging sustainable lifestyle changes. The HEEL program has roots in three entities: the land grant system, the Cooperative Extension Service (CES), and University of Kentucky Academic Health Centers. The land grant system, created in 1862, provided public lands to establish colleges focused on agriculture, home economics, and mechanical arts. As an implementation of the Smith-Lever Act of 1914, the U.S. Department of Agriculture created the CES in order to "extend" research and expertise from land-grant universities to ordinary citizens. Counties are the typical unit of service distribution within the states with this system; as will be described below, extension agents operate in all 120 counties of Kentucky.

The initial objective of the CES was to address the work and family issues of rural/agricultural residents; as such, it focused on advancements in farm technology and home economics. As farm life evolved, however, new challenges arose for rural residents, including occupational hazards, substance abuse, and chronic disease. As these health issues began to be added to the CES agenda, the need for a partnership with various academic health centers (AHCs) became apparent. The AHC is typically a group of health profession schools offering training in medicine, public health, dentistry, and nursing. The University of Kentucky is one of few universities with an AHC and a College of Agriculture (with an embedded CES) on the same campus, an arrangement that facilitates communication and collaboration. HEEL is the result of a formal partnership between the College of Agriculture (and the CES it sponsors) and the Colleges of Nursing, Public Health, and other health care disciplines.

Vision and Purpose

HEEL serves as a catalyst for change by bridging people, resources, ideas, and actions, and generally leveraging the unique land grant system. This provides a foundation for health outreach and education, augmented by university-based research and formal collaborations with other long-term partners.

The formation of core collaborations within the University of Kentucky was the key to the development of HEEL; naturally, this type of integration required substantial "buy-in" from the university administration. In 2001, the year of HEEL's inception, a new president – Lee T. Todd Jr – took office at the University of Kentucky. He articulated a bold vision for his administration: "We need to have a higher purpose in our approach. It's taking the Kentucky uglies – the low literacy, poor health, low income – and having a higher purpose to say: 'Let's look at the things that have held Kentucky back and see how we can help.'"

Addressing these conditions is an important component of the University of Kentucky's goal of becoming a "top 20" public research institution by 2020; HEEL is a significant cornerstone of the strategy to accomplish this. President Todd, a former business executive, recognized a special resource and opportunity in the extensive statewide network of the CES. As a "communications system with few rivals for efficiency and effectiveness," it offered a platform to deliver health information to all Kentuckians.

The purpose of HEEL is an elaboration of the Healthy People 2010 national framework for prevention. The objectives include the following:

- To educate and empower individuals and families to adopt healthy behaviours and lifestyles
- To build community capacity to improve health
- To educate consumers to make informed health choices

There continues to be a strong commitment to the family, true to the roots of the CES. Debbie Murray, the associate director of HEEL and a key informant for this section of the book, stated that family is "the first place where health begins." This sentiment is reflected in the number of programs pursued by extension agents that are aimed at the well-being of the family and the communities in which they live. Although individual behaviour change is certainly important, the community perspective means that the strategies involved are much broader.

Organization

There are over 700 professional extension personnel located in country offices that are sponsored by the University of Kentucky. Two positions are key to the HEEL program: the cooperative extension agent (CEA) and the health extension specialist. HEEL services are primarily delivered by CEAs based out of county offices. Although the original CEAs were trained in family and consumer sciences, they now have varying educational backgrounds, from bachelors' degrees to PhDs, and in areas ranging from health and social sciences to fine arts. Along with the broad spectrum of knowledge found on CEA teams, there is a consistent base of expertise in community education as a core competency.

In addition to specific program delivery and evaluation (see below), CEAs facilitate local coalitions to identify community health needs and available resources. CEAs are also instrumental in identifying and

Figure 7.1. Map of Kentucky.

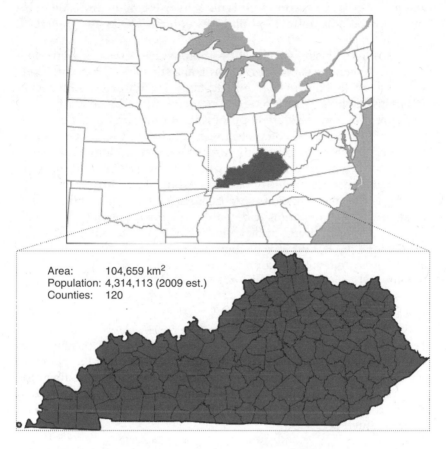

Area: 104,659 km^2
Population: 4,314,113 (2009 est.)
Counties: 120

training lay opinion leaders to promote and/or reinforce programs. Reports suggest that this approach has been very successful. When local, respected members of the community deliver culturally appropriate messages, there is more "buy-in" from neighbours and friends. This aspect of HEEL is deeply rooted in the "diffusion of innovations" theory. The originator of the theory, Everett Rogers, defined diffusion as "the process by which an innovation is communicated through certain channels over time among the members of a social system." Interestingly, Rogers's educational background was in agriculture and rural sociology, leading to a 47-year academic career during which he published numerous books on communication networks and health information campaigns. With this pedigree, it is not surprising that "diffusion of innovations" became an integral part of Kentucky's CES and the HEEL program.

The health extension specialist position, which serves as a link specifically between the College of Nursing and the HEEL program, is one of the first of its kind in the United States. Health extension specialists act in the capacity of a program manager for CEAs, ensuring that HEEL programs are delivered appropriately, program impact data collected, and evaluations completed in a timely way. As noted above, they work closely with university researchers in adapting existing programs or developing new ones. They have many other responsibilities, including: managing new program development and implementation; serving as the major resource person for CEAs by providing a variety of educational materials and health bulletins; assisting CEAs with displays, demonstrations, and presentations at health fairs; and being advocates of the importance of community-based health extension by serving on state-level advisory committees addressing topics such as diabetes and obesity.

Targeted HEEL Initiatives

Statewide, numerous programs have been developed in partnership with HEEL across a broad spectrum of health conditions; the planning process has involved many colleges and academic departments at the University of Kentucky. Collaborative efforts have ultimately yielded over 1,770 health education and health promotion programs. Several are highlighted below.

DIABETES PARTNERSHIP

According to Murray, the associate director, the majority of HEEL's initiatives are "focused on the two things where every person can make a difference – their personal health in regards to managing their weight and their level of physical activity." Motivating individuals to make lifestyle changes is a common theme in the various initiatives. Pike County's effort to reduce diabetes rates provides one example. Pike County is the largest county in the area development district (ADD) of Kentucky that has the state's highest obesity rate and is the least physically active – two major risk factors for diabetes. The ADD in question was also ranked first out of the state's 15 districts in terms of diabetes-related mortality.

As a member of the Pike County Diabetes Partnership, the county's Cooperative Extension Service office has been actively encouraging people to incorporate healthy eating habits and physical activity into their daily routines. Diabetes cooking schools and the development of walking paths are two examples of the local efforts. The cooking schools, taught by extension agents and local health departments, cover topics such as recipe adaptation and counting carbohydrates for improving blood sugar levels. Cristy Honaker, the Pike County family and consumer sciences extension agent, noted that class graduates have changed the way they prepare meals, incorporated physical activity into their daily lives, and generally improved their blood sugar control. Many participants also lost weight and experienced an increase in energy.

The CES has also helped to develop four walking paths around the city of Pikeville, the county seat of Pike County. "The walking paths provide an opportunity to motivate community members to get out and explore the area," Honaker said. Each trail varies in location, length, and difficulty; the intention of the overall project is to motivate residents to try new walking routes and to increase their walking time. According to Honaker, the Diabetes Partnership hopes to develop similar walking paths in other communities in Pike County.

GET MOVING KENTUCKY!

As a result of Kentucky's 2003 ranking as lowest in the nation for physical activity among adults, the Get Moving Kentucky! initiative was launched. HEEL project staff developed this outreach campaign in partnership with the University of Kentucky Wellness Center and the Kentucky Cabinet for Health Services. The Get Moving Kentucky! program focuses on increasing the physical activity of Kentuckians while acknowledging the effects of low socioeconomic status and limited resources. During development of the program, extension agents held focus groups, and feedback was received indicating that a physical activity program focusing on one type of activity (e.g., walking) would not be appropriate for all counties of Kentucky. Suitable and safe areas for walking are not always available, especially in rural or remote regions. One solution is to multiply the "pathways" of physical activity enhancement.

Get Moving Kentucky! uses just such a multipronged approach. It includes an 8-week physical activity program combined with other health lessons, as well as a web-based tracking system that allows participants to record their physical activity progress. Participants earn

Physical Activity Miles (PAMs); one PAM is equal to 15 minutes of activity. Importantly, all activities count and are translated into a PAM equivalent – including gardening, dancing, and house cleaning. Participants are encouraged to "earn" two PAMs every day over the 8-week program. By setting achievable goals and means for all Kentuckians, the program shows that engaging in physical activity for better health is within reach, despite low socioeconomic status and other barriers to accessing physical activity resources.

Get Moving Kentucky! has several other components, including encouraging communities to form a task force to develop a year-round physical activity plan; providing extension agents with a curriculum that covers physical activity issues such as safety, weight management, and other benefits related to chronic disease; and mounting a major media awareness campaign. Between 2004 and 2007, over 230,000 people across the state were reached by CEAs incorporating elements of Get Moving Kentucky!

LITERACY, EATING AND ACTIVITY FOR PRIMARY YOUTH HEALTH

Literacy, Eating and Activity for Primary Youth Health (LEAP) is a series of 22 storybook-based lessons to teach children about being physically active; eating more fruits and vegetables, low-fat dairy products, and whole grains; and otherwise being healthy. The program was developed by HEEL in partnership with the Kentucky Cardiovascular Coalition and the Kentucky Department of Education. As with other HEEL work, LEAP is being coordinated through county cooperative extension service offices in each county. Delivery, however, is not limited to CEAs; public librarians, child care consultants, and family resource centre coordinators have also attended training sessions and implemented the program. In 2009, 78 Kentucky counties offered LEAP, reaching 16,647 children aged 3–8 years; evaluation suggested that 76% of the participating children increased their physical activity.

Kentucky Cancer Program

History and Mission

The Kentucky Cancer Program (KCP) demonstrates an approach that has remarkable parallels with HEEL. It is a cancer prevention and control network established in 1982 by the Kentucky General Assembly, and now nationally recognized in the United States as a model for

Figure 7.2. Map of Kentucky by Area Development District (ADD) and Component Counties.

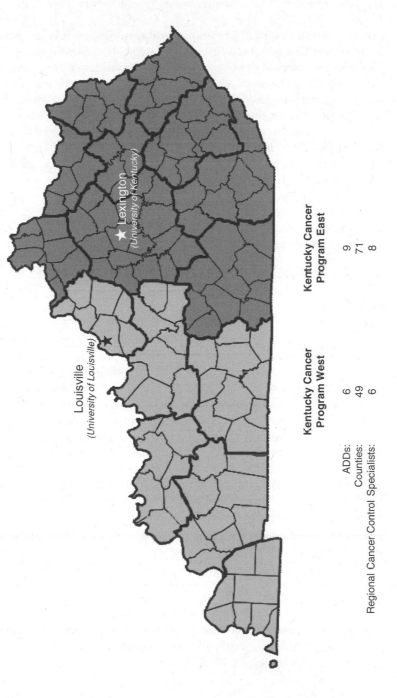

Louisville
(University of Louisville)

Lexington
(University of Kentucky)

	Kentucky Cancer Program West	Kentucky Cancer Program East
ADDs:	6	9
Counties:	49	71
Regional Cancer Control Specialists:	6	8

cancer control. The KCP is a unique program in that it is state-funded, university-affiliated, and community-based. It is jointly administered by Cancer Centers at the University of Louisville and the University of Kentucky. This strong academic connection, similar to that described for HEEL, enables KCP activities to be evidence-based, driven by up-to-date cancer data, and integrated with research efforts.

KCP's mission is to reduce cancer incidence and mortality in all of Kentucky's 120 counties by promoting and coordinating cancer education, research, and service programs. The four major goals of the KCP are as follows:

- To increase awareness of cancer prevention and risk factors
- To increase cancer screenings and early detection
- To increase access to state-of-the-art cancer treatment and care resources
- To improve the quality of life for cancer survivors

Organization

The KCP operates via a network of 14 cancer control specialists in regional offices; these specialists provide leadership on cancer prevention and control initiatives geared to each of Kentucky's counties. The counties are grouped into 15 area development districts (ADDs); there is generally one cancer control specialist assigned to each ADD. Each ADD has a district cancer council (DCC) with a membership comprised of various professional health-related disciplines (medicine, nursing, social work, etc.); staff from organizations such as the Cooperative Extension Service, the American Cancer Society, and local public health departments; and members of the general public and the cohort of cancer survivors in the area. The DCCs provide a common forum for cancer control partners to network, coordinate, and collaborate. KCP works closely with the 15 DCCs to share cancer data, focus interventions and strategies on priority cancers and at-risk populations, mobilize resources, and ultimately evaluate the impact of intervention activities. Cancer control specialists are instrumental in establishing and maintaining the DCC in their region; together with the DCCs, they are considered the backbone of KCP.

The KCP is closely integrated with the cancer control programs of the two universities. This is reflected in the activities of the cancer control specialists, including:

- Bringing cancer control expertise to communities and health care providers through workshops, conferences, training, and academic detailing ("detailing" is a format originated by pharmaceutical company representatives of offering brief, focused training to physicians and other staff in primary care settings)
- Facilitating community-based research initiatives
- Representing the pertinent Cancer Center on advisory boards, committees, and coalitions within the community
- Facilitating joint planning and communication between community and university representatives

One of the key informants for this section of the book was Kathy Rack, a senior Regional Cancer Control Specialist for the Kentucky Cancer Program (East). She noted that a key element of her job description involves community assessment. Using comprehensive data related to demographics, health status, and cancer rates, such specialists endeavour to understand the composition of a community and the issues it faces. They present an annual "community report card" to the district cancer council, allowing cancer issues and service gaps to be identified. This information has direct impacts on education planning for KCP and is also very important for the community partners in determining how their programs will be targeted and implemented. Once gaps are identified, best practices for addressing them are then determined at the DCC level. Organizations are sometimes reluctant to adopt best practices, as they have limited knowledge or experience of program effectiveness. To facilitate adoption of best practice interventions, the KCP conducts pilot or demonstration projects to model how they operate and develop evidence of their impact. Once effectiveness is proven, the program is more enthusiastically taken up by other organizations, with ongoing support from KCP. KCP is then able to transfer its energies to other areas where gaps exist (see Figure 7.3).

Another facet of the cancer control specialist role involves recruiting and training lay health educators. Recently, a cervical cancer screening demonstration project was implemented, in which the cancer control specialist worked with *promotoras* (Spanish-speaking Latina community health workers) and African-American coalitions to increase cervical cancer screening rates in their communities. The often hard-to-reach target populations – low-income, minority women aged 40–64 – received home visits from the lay health educators. As well, media reports through the radio and newspapers were used to promote the

Figure 7.3. Innovation Cycle.

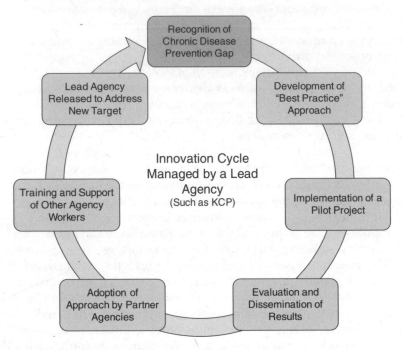

value of screening. The project was very successful, and highlighted a creative and effective way of reaching into these communities.

Targeted KCP Initiatives

KCP's commitment to fighting cancer through education, service, collaboration, and research is demonstrated by the wide range of initiatives undertaken to address cancer prevention and control needs in the state. KCP sponsors cancer screenings, awareness campaigns, survivor support services, community-based research, and public and professional education, among other efforts. Some of the major initiatives are outlined below.

COOPER/CLAYTON METHOD TO STOP SMOKING

KCP collaborates with local health departments and other partners to train people from across the state to facilitate Cooper/Clayton Method to Stop Smoking classes in their communities. Cooper/Clayton is a 13-week program combining weekly classes, peer support, and nicotine replacement therapy. KCP has been coordinating the program since 2000 in partnership with its developers Richard Clayton, PhD, and Thomas Cooper, DDS. Reflecting the innovation cycle described above (see Figure 7.3), KCP has trained more than 1,250 facilitators from a variety of agencies in the method. KCP also offers refresher courses so facilitators can keep up to date with new resources and the latest research on smoking cessation.

ASPIRE

Studies have shown that a majority of Kentucky youths who use tobacco want to quit, but there are few cessation programs designed for them. KCP collaborated in the autumn of 2009 with 12 middle and high schools in three area development districts to test a new program for youths called *A Smoking Prevention Interactive Experience* (ASPIRE). The interactive Internet-based program incorporates colourful animation and videos. Kentucky is one of 14 states to pilot-test the program, and the only state to test it as part of a funded research study. The study involved 1,035 Grade 7 and Grade 10 students. In the first school term, KCP cancer control specialists surveyed the students on tobacco use and attitudes before their exposure to ASPIRE. KCP will follow up with the students in the spring of 2010 to determine whether the program made a difference in the students' tobacco use, attitudes, and attempts to quit. ASPIRE was developed by researchers at the University of Texas M.D. Anderson Cancer Center, with funding from the National Cancer Institute and the George and Barbara Bush Foundation.

HORSES AND HOPE

The second annual Horses and Hope campaign was conducted in the summer and fall of 2009 at four thoroughbred race tracks in Kentucky. The campaign sponsored a Pink Race Day at each track, where fans received breast cancer information in their racing programs, visited breast cancer educational displays, and watched a race dedicated to the disease (with horses wearing pink saddlecloths). Breast cancer survivors who purchased advance tickets received gifts and educational materials at registration, had their photo taken with Kentucky's First Lady, enjoyed a buffet luncheon, and sat together in a reserved section of the grandstand. Horses and Hope also included Education and Screening Days, where female track workers and female relatives of male track workers received one-on-one breast cancer education from bilingual staff and free mammograms through an on-site van. Most participants had no health insurance, and would not have been screened were it not for the program. The following results were obtained by Horses and Hope activities during the past 2 years: 146,844 Kentucky racing fans were exposed to breast cancer awareness messages; 3,517 survivors were supported at Pink Race Days; and 1,119 female track workers or relatives of male track workers were educated about breast cancer, with 213 of those actually being screened.

Case Analysis

This section will consider how the role of the extension agents/cancer control specialists and the context of the Kentucky programs compare with, and offer a perspective on, the CPE program in British Columbia.

Parallels with British Columbia and the CPE Program

As introduced in chapter 3, both examples of regional health staff in Kentucky, extension agents and cancer control specialists, demonstrate important overlaps with CPEs in British Columbia. This includes the generalist prevention role endorsed by each organization, with efforts that are filtered through a community engagement approach within a defined population. Among the case studies in this book, the KCP offers what is perhaps the closest match to British Columbia's community-based prevention educator program. The most obvious parallel is that they are both focused on cancer prevention. About 90% of the activities of KCP are related to primary prevention and screening of cancer, with the remainder focusing on treatment issues. Most other programs examined in this book have a broader agenda, dealing with other chronic disease such as diabetes and heart disease, or with health promotion in a more generalized way.

Second, the number and type of staff in the two programs demonstrate a close overlap. KCP has 15 cancer control specialists assigned to specific regions of the state; the CPE program has 20 CPEs covering specific areas throughout the province. Both the CPEs and the cancer control specialists are professionals who live and work in the communities they serve. They work independently, yet are part of a team that occasionally meets together; sometimes two or more staff members work together on the same project.

The main focus of both HEEL and the CPE program involves addressing disease risk factors. Although the CPEs are specifically assigned to the cancer prevention arena, there are strong overlaps between cancer risk factors and those associated with other major chronic diseases. Smoking cessation, nutrition, and physical activity are thus key targets of both programs. A major goal of HEEL is to have an impact on the "Kentucky uglies" – one of which is high cancer rates. Kentucky has the highest rate of cancer deaths in the United States, at 211 per 100,000, compared to the national average of 181.

The role of the CPE has been described in terms of being a catalyst, a motivator, and a collaborator. In an interview with the associate director of HEEL, the term "catalyst" was also used to characterize HEEL's extension agents. Although it includes some service delivery, the role of the extension agent is more involved with building a supportive community. The aim is to create an environment where people will be inspired to take up programs that will help them to make changes in their lives. This perfectly matches the philosophy behind the British Columbia program, as described by one of the CPEs: "We provide information and tools for people/organizations/communities to make smarter, healthier choices for themselves, particularly when it comes to cancer prevention. We can point them in a good direction, motivate them to take the steps necessary to make the changes in their organizations/communities/lives, and enlist the help of other groups and organizations to make it possible."

Having pre-existing connections in the assigned region is a key requirement of the CPE role, forming a foundation on which to forge new strategic relationships. In short, having local people "delivering the message" is seen to be foundational to the program. Similarly, the extension agents, cancer control specialists, and the lay opinion leaders in Kentucky are all community-based, with many personal and/or professional linkages in their regions. As may be expected with a program that has century-old roots in every county, the existing HEEL relationships can be very long-term. Interestingly, the sense of community trust sometimes is extended beyond the individuals to the position itself. The result is that, even when there is staff turnover, less of the incoming agent's time and energy has to be spent on building the confidence of a network. Most of the KCP cancer control specialists have held their positions for 10 years or more; they have a history with the communities they serve and are therefore accepted as trustworthy. The low staff turnover rate is indicative of the staff commitment to the KCP and passion for the work they do.

Improvements in health outcomes such as cancer incidence and mortality may take many years due to the phenomenon of disease latency, although the effect of some risk factor change on certain chronic diseases can be seen much earlier. Fortunately, regardless of the disease in view, changes in risky behaviours can be measurable over a shorter term. In the past decade, Kentucky has seen substantial improvements in certain risk factors. For instance, the prevalence of smoking has decreased from 30% of adults to 25%, and the proportion of adults who are physically active has increased from 57% to almost 70%. The prevalence of obesity, however, has been consistently rising, similar to the experience of many jurisdictions around the world. The general risk factor pattern is similar in British Columbia, although in Kentucky it started and ended with lower absolute rates. From 1994 to 2005, the prevalence of smoking in the province dropped by 30%, from 21.6% to 15.2% of people aged 20 years and older. The prevalence of obesity, on the other hand, increased by 25% over the same period, from 7.7% to 9.6%. In contrast to Kentucky's ranking in the United States, the absolute rates of these risk factors in British Columbia over the decade have consistently remained the lowest in Canada.

Attributing the observed improvements in smoking and physical inactivity to a specific program is difficult, given the multiple simultaneous initiatives in the state of Kentucky, but the trends are undoubtedly encouraging to managers and workers in HEEL and the KCP. The CPEs in British Columbia also expressed a desire to know whether the work they are doing is making a difference; while they may know of stories of behaviour changes in clients influenced by their efforts, it is important to track the developments across a defined population. This calls for a timely and accurate risk factor surveillance system. Similar to the situation in Kentucky, even good risk factor information in British Columbia would not automatically prove the effectiveness of any one program, but it would be suggestive of the value of the overall strategic efforts.

Contrasts with British Columbia and the CPE Program

On the surface, a significant difference between HEEL and the CPEs involves the program sizes. The population of the state of Kentucky, at 4.2 million, is similar to that of British Columbia, but the land area of British Columbia is approximately nine times greater. This underlines the differential in HEEL capacity, with its over 700 full-time personnel spread across Kentucky; by comparison there are about 20 contracted, part-time CPEs in British Columbia. Debbie Murray, associate director of HEEL, stressed that no health budget in the contemporary world could ever reproduce this type of program and its existing network. Although the HEEL strategy per se is relatively new, it is built on a foundation of university-connected, community-based workers that has been in place for nearly a century. Despite ranking 37th in the United States by area, Kentucky has the third-highest number of counties, at 120. These subdivisions were originally created based on the distance that could be travelled by horseback in a single day, similar to the history of municipal boundary-setting in Finland. Some Kentucky counties are less than 200 square miles in area; the largest is Pike County, at 788 square miles. Many have a population of less than 20,000. In every county, an office was established many decades ago for the cooperative extension service – the foundation on which HEEL is built. The challenge for the CPE program lies in reaching the same population base as Kentucky's, but in certain cases spread over much larger areas; when this is combined with the mountainous topography, the northern climate, and the isolation of some communities, the reproducibility of the HEEL program is further called into question.

As discussed above, there is substantial overlap between HEEL and the CPE program with regard to the risk factors that are addressed. HEEL, however, ultimately delves into a wider range of health-related issues, well beyond the typical limits of cancer prevention work. Of course, in this way it also differs from the narrower focus of the other statewide program, the KCP. Agriculture was the basis of the cooperative extension service when it was first established in the early 1900s, and it still plays an important role in the work of the extension agents. Food security and food safety are significant issues of the modern age. Private and community gardens have greatly increased in popularity; the urban gardening and local food movements are examples of agriculture-related work occupying the extension agents in Kentucky. Other programming may help people to develop skills in accessing affordable nutritious food and knowledge of food-safe practices. These areas draw on expertise from another university faculty that has deep roots with the extension program, namely, Family and Consumer Sciences. Extension agents with this background promote healthy families and communities by encouraging physical activity and good nutrition, and also through educational programs on topics such as parenting skills, money management, and generally making good lifestyle decisions.

The multifaceted academic connection that is a crucial part of the success of HEEL and KCP is not found to the same extent in the CPE program, although the latter may benefit from the world-class research resources of the British Columbia Cancer Agency. KCP, being jointly administered by cancer centres at the two leading universities in the state, is deeply rooted in the world of postsecondary education and investigation. According to the KCP East Director Debra Armstrong, the close relationship with researchers is central to the program's success; among other benefits, it lends a high degree of credibility and gravitas to the cancer control specialists. Likewise, HEEL's development was spearheaded by the University of Kentucky's president, and all specialist HEEL personnel are direct employees of the university. Perhaps most important, though, is the connection that has been forged between the cooperative extension agents, who are partners with HEEL, and various university researchers. This critical communication channel has resulted in the development of locally adapted, community-oriented programming that is also evidence-based. This instils confidence in risk factor messaging and other interventions. Among other partnership possibilities, the fact that the College of Agriculture and its cooperative extension service are located on the same campus as the Academic Health Centre provides for many synergies.

Insights for the CPE (and Similar) Programs

A network of cancer prevention agents reaching every region is valuable. In this respect, the KCP and CPEs may represent a best practice scenario to which other cancer-specific programs may aspire when the aim is reaching an entire population with prevention messages and other initiatives. Although the resources that would be required to establish a network similar to the cooperative extension service in Kentucky are unrealistic, the KCP model represents a scaled-down version and may be more widely applicable.

Risk factor reduction should be embedded in a broader perspective on health. Reducing risk factors by focusing on targets such as nutrition, physical activity, and tobacco use is a large part of both the KCP and HEEL, with the ultimate goal of reducing cancer and chronic diseases, respectively. HEEL, however, adopts a more holistic view of health. There is a recognition that health may be defined as a broad sense of well-being that begins with the family; thus, HEEL takes into account the social aspects of an individual's needs, and embraces both psychological and physical outcomes. Furthermore, there are many factors outside of the individual realm that play a significant role in shaping one's quality of life; these include social determinants such as unemployment and poverty, which require advocacy and ultimately a response at the policy level. Although direct advocacy is not an appropriate role for state employees, HEEL indirectly addresses social factors by, for instance, operating programs that focus on empowering community leaders.

Sustained commitment is one key to program success. There really is no substitute for longevity in the community. An organization such as the British Columbia Cancer Agency prevention department and its CPE program must commit to "stay the course" in order to have the kind of impact that is desired. When it can be achieved, the longevity of individual staff members is also very important. The social networks built over time by HEEL and the KCP are considered critical to the respective programs. Any successes are strongly aligned with continuity and longevity, according to KCP East Director Debra Armstrong. It is likely that, as the CPE program continues to develop, building relationships will be less time-consuming, because there will already be a significant network in place.

Continuing the theme introduced in the previous point, a deep community connection is critical. A foundational component of the CPE program, HEEL, and the KCP is the connection of the agents to the communities in which they work. Not only do they both live and work in the communities they serve, but they are often well connected through various community organizations, opinion leaders, and groups. Such a network is necessary for facilitating their work in mobilizing the community to improve health. In addition, when the agent is a known and respected member of the community, there is much more credence attached to the messages they are trying to convey. Both HEEL and KCP have taken this a step further by enlisting the help of lay opinion leaders, by all accounts a successful component of their strategy. Further encouragement to consider adding lay opinion leaders as an intentional approach may be found in the context of North Carolina (see the next chapter).

Fostering a strong partnership with the academic/research world brings great benefits. Foundational to HEEL and KCP is the deep connection with academics and researchers; HEEL is in fact an extension of the University of Kentucky, and KCP is also based at that institution and at the University of Louisville. More important than any formal institutional home is the fact that both programs are intentionally structured so that there is open two-way communication between field agents and university researchers. This arrangement would generate advantages for any similar program, including: access to information about community needs; up-to-date knowledge about evidence-based interventions that can be adapted to local situations; and high credibility for agents that helps to foster "buy-in" from local organizations, leaders, and clients.

Evaluation challenges exist in every prevention setting. Unlike the unique experience of the North Karelia Project, which launched essentially in an environment devoid of any other substantial prevention activity, the work of the CPEs in British Columbia does not occur in isolation. As in Kentucky and other industrialized settings in the world, there are many health-promoting organizations at work in British Columbia. Attributing short-term behaviour change or long-term health outcomes to any single program is a complex task.

Conclusion

There are limits to how far and fast a prevention program may expand. However, there are encouragements in the Kentucky story that might drive cancer prevention programming much further. Budgets are a limitation that must be overcome in every jurisdiction, of course, but so is lack of imagination.

As suggested above, HEEL stands apart from the CPE program in terms of its deep roots in the land and agriculture. Certain B.C. CPEs may be involved with discussions and planning around food security, but it is difficult to match the historic momentum of such matters within the cooperative extension service. There is no doubt that building on the connection between agriculture and health makes sense. As noted by Gillespie and colleagues of the International Food Policy Research Institute in Washington, DC:

> Agriculture is fundamental for good health through the production of the world's food, fiber and materials for shelter, and in some systems, medicinal plants. Among rural communities, it contributes to livelihoods and food security, and provides income which can be spent on health care and prevention. Yet agriculture is associated with many of the world's major health problems, including undernutrition, malaria, AIDS, foodborne diseases, diet-related chronic diseases, and a range of occupational health hazards.

As fuel costs, environmental concerns, the "eat local" movement, and desire for organic produce continue to shape individual and community food choices, the integration of health and agriculture is likely to intensify in Kentucky, British Columbia, and beyond.

Sources and Further Reading

The Cooper/Clayton Method to Stop Smoking. Available at http://www. stopsmoking4ever.org (accessed 12 February 2010).

Kentucky Cancer Program. *A Unique Cancer Control Program - 2006–2008 Biennial Report.* 2009. Available at http://www.kycancerprogram.org/ (accessed July 2011).

Lee DS, Chiu M, Manuel DG, et al, and the Canadian Cardiovascular Outcomes Research Team. Trends in risk factors for cardiovascular disease in Canada: temporal, socio-demographic and geographic factors. CMAJ. 2009;181(3-4):E55–66. http://dx.doi.org/10.1503/cmaj.081629. Medline:19620271

Literacy, Eating, and Activity for Primary Youth Health (LEAP). Overview and planning materials. Available at http://www.ca.uky.edu/HES/fcs/heel/leap/overview_and_planning_materials.pdf (accessed 8 April 2010).

Riley P. Collaboration for prevention of chronic disease in Kentucky: the Health Education through Extension Leaders (HEEL) program. Nurs Clin North Am. 2008;43(3):329–40, vii. http://dx.doi.org/10.1016/j.cnur.2008.04.007. Medline:18674667

U.S. National Vital Statistics Report. April 17, 2009. Available at http://www.cdc.gov/nchs/data/nvsr/nvsr57/nvsr57_14.pdf (accessed 23 January 2010).

8 North Carolina: Community Health Ambassadors

As she left her weekly quilting group, Rosemary had a great feeling of accomplishment – and it had nothing to do with quilting. One of the group members had started a regular walking routine; another had tried a new recipe that was a healthier version of an old favourite; a third had signed up for a stop-smoking class. Rosemary knew that these changes had come about because she had started talking with them about the importance of good nutrition and physical activity, giving them ideas for simple changes they could make to improve their health. She had recently completed the Community Health Ambassador (CHA) training program and was eager to share her newfound knowledge with friends and family. At first, when her pastor had suggested she become a CHA, she did not think she could do it. Rosemary did not feel that she was a leader, and she did not like public speaking. But she soon learned that as a CHA she only needed to spread the health message among her usual social circle. With her involvement in church activities, through quilting, on school council, and with her extended family, that social circle was surprisingly large. Rosemary was determined to reach as many as she could to help them with diabetes management and lifestyle changes – and she knew one of the best ways to do that was to be an example. As part of her CHA training, she had signed a health pledge agreement; since then, she had improved her own diet and incorporated exercise into her daily routine. These are important steps to diabetes prevention and overall better health, and are a key part of the message that needed to be conveyed. As she walked home that evening, Rosemary was sure that other feelings of accomplishment were just around the corner.

The Community Health Ambassador Program (CHAP) was developed recently in North Carolina to engage community leaders in helping to eliminate health disparities. It involves multiple partnerships with local health departments, community- and faith-based organizations, and the community college system. The initial focus of CHAP was on improving diabetes awareness, management, and prevention.

Technically, the true parallel with the CPE program in British Columbia is not the lay health ambassadors per se, but the professional or lay supervisors of groups of ambassadors in different areas. However, as will be discussed below, the program is still valuable in the present context as an example of one strategic way that leaders such as the CPEs could pursue a cancer prevention agenda on a regionalized basis.

Background

The state of North Carolina has long been supportive of community-based approaches to the prevention and control of chronic disease. In 1986, the statewide North Carolina Health Promotion Program was developed to provide resources to local health departments. Its aim was to encourage the development of community-based interventions to increase physical activity, healthy eating, and tobacco cessation. Among other efforts, a renewed focus on policy and environmental changes to address prevention of chronic disease in the past decade has dramatically increased local health department reports of population-level improvements. Other mechanisms of change have been a substantial expansion of health outreach to targeted minority populations and implementation of such programs in various community settings. Branded campaigns such as Charlotte REACH 2010 and Project DIRECT are examples of successful, community-level strategies for chronic disease prevention and management; these were specifically focused on diabetes in the African-American population.

CHAP differs from other North Carolina community-based health promotion projects in that it is a statewide effort that uses trained community members to deliver health education messages rather than traditional volunteers. The North Carolina Office of Minority Health and Health Disparities (NCOMHHD) developed CHAP in 2006, based on the following objectives:

• To identify local perspectives, priorities, and solutions regarding common, challenging public health issues disproportionately affecting racial or ethnic minority populations, such as type 2 diabetes
• To enhance knowledge about the community's health concerns

Figure 8.1. Map of North Carolina.

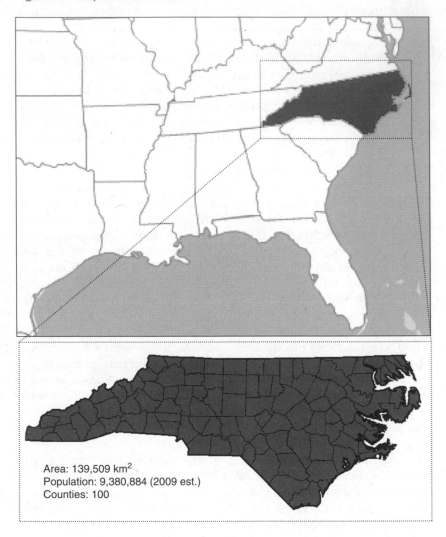

Area: 139,509 km^2
Population: 9,380,884 (2009 est.)
Counties: 100

- To increase the community's ability to access existing health and human services, programs, and resources
- To develop a network of health care advocates throughout the state

Diabetes had an overall 9.3% prevalence rate in North Carolina in 2008. Ethnic and minority populations are disproportionately affected by the disease. In 2008, African Americans had the highest diabetes prevalence rate in the state, at 15.6%, followed by Native Americans at 12.4%. CHAP addresses this sort of disparity in a number of ways, beginning by forming partnerships with various organizations that represent minority population groups (described below). Of course, the strategy begins with ensuring that CHAs are recruited from within the target population.

Since CHAP was implemented, over 300 community health ambassadors (CHAs) from 17 counties have been trained. As Figure 8.1 indicates, this means that further expansion among counties in the state is certainly possible and desirable. The initial focus of CHAP has been on diabetes awareness, prevention, and management; CHA community activities include one-on-one dissemination of diabetes self-management tips, diabetes talks to small groups, and recruitment of family members, friends, and neighbours to sign healthy living pledges. It is important to realize that these initiatives are meant to spread within natural affinity circles and generally within close physical proximity to the CHA. A recipient of a health message may very well be a relative, a friend, and a neighbour all at the same time.

Partnerships

Prior to the implementation of CHAP, the NCOMHHD engaged in multiple local and statewide partnerships and collaborations. These are considered a key reason for the general success of its efforts, and the foundations for the eventual establishment of CHAP. Examples of these partnerships are listed below:

Success Dynamics Community Development Corporation (SDCDC) – A faith-based, non-profit organization providing preventive education and access to medical care for minority residents. The SDCDC executive director serves as the statewide coordinator for CHAP, initially identifying pilot areas where CHAs could be recruited and trained.

Old North State Medical Society – An association of African-American physicians. The society recruited local physicians to train the student CHAs on the clinical aspects of diabetes.

Faith-based Organizations (FBOs) and Community-based Organizations – Their memberships represented pools from which to recruit CHAs; they also provide meeting space for workshops, training sessions, and screening programs.

American Indian Tribes – Their memberships represented pools from which to recruit CHAs.

North Carolina Community College System (NCCCS) – Supports CHAP training by providing instructors for courses and providing continuing education credits to all CHA trainees who successfully complete the course requirements.

University of North Carolina at Greensboro Nursing Program – Donates resources to CHAP, such as diabetes testing equipment, medical supplies, and other materials used in the CHA training.

Local Health Departments – Serve as referral agencies for health concerns identified by CHAs working in communities, and provide health educational materials and resources.

Recruitment and Training

Key CHAP partner organizations, as outlined above, were asked to identify and recruit trusted community members to be trained as CHAs. One such partner, a collaboration of FBOs known as the Community Empowerment Network, enthusiastically endorsed the project, and pastors from the network preregistered for CHA training. In fact, ministers from different denominations continue to assist CHAP by promoting and advertising the program.

The involvement of churches in health education programs in the United States is becoming increasingly popular for a variety of reasons. The majority of Americans attend a church; in North Carolina, part of the historic Bible belt, over 90% of adults report some kind of religious affiliation. This makes the church a prime foundation from which a large sector of the population is accessible. As well, churches tend to have appropriate resources for organized health promotion activities, including meeting rooms and kitchens. Some churches in North Carolina and other parts of the United States have integrated physical and spiritual concerns to such an extent that community health outreach has become an official part of their mission. They are thus very open to promoting CHAP, hosting related health promotion activities, and even participating in research studies.

The passionate collaboration described above, along with a supportive network of complementary organizations, was instrumental in achieving a high recruitment rate across the state; a remarkable 146 CHAs were recruited and trained in the initial 18-month launch phase.

Requirements to be considered a CHA trainee include:

- An expressed interest in learning more about health issues
- Willingness to volunteer for 2 years
- Demonstration of some leadership qualities

Recruits, once confirmed as suitable candidates, registered for CHAP's training program. This 20-hour course was delivered over a 2-week period by NCCCS instructors. It consisted of classroom instruction, interactive sessions, and field practice. Course components focused on awareness, health promotion, and disease prevention strategies, as well as approaches to identifying and accessing existing health care services and resources. The field project involved collecting of information on health programs that could be included in a local directory.

On successful completion of the training course, students received 2.0 continuing education credits from their local community college. As a further requirement for graduation from CHAP and deployment in the community, students signed a pledge indicating their commitment to do the following:

1 Engage in healthier lifestyles to improve their own health
2 Participate in at least one Success Dynamics-sponsored continuing education session
3 Complete their local resource directory
4 "Translate" health information to at least 100 people within the first year after graduation

This pledge was meant to ensure that each CHA not only performed the duties of the position, but also acted as a role model in healthy living. The continuing education component is important in encouraging ongoing participation in the program. Maintaining a high retention rate and seeing CHAs commit beyond the initial 2 years are vital to the long-term success of the program. Although external incentives are likely only going to be a small part of CHA retention, they can be symbolically useful. CHAP graduates in the first wave were awarded a $50 stipend from Success Dynamics for successful completion of the training.

Success and Sustainability

As seen most clearly in the North Karelia Project, evaluation and monitoring of a program are often pivotal to its longevity, recalibration (as required), and ongoing success. In the case of CHAP, feedback from the CHAs led to key changes in the program in order to enhance its sustainability. Besides the in-training evaluations conducted as part of the NCCCS course, further information was gathered from 100 CHAs via a mailed assessment tool. The purpose of the tool was to identify the types of outreach activities provided by CHAs, the additional training and support needs of the CHAs, and the successes and challenges they had experienced to date. In keeping with the tradition of recognizing special service rendered, a modest stipend was provided to those who returned the completed assessment to the evaluators.

Assessment Strategy

Results from the mailed assessment indicated that over 90% of the CHAs were interested in continuing their work. In most of the comments, CHAs indicated that they were enthusiastic about the program, especially with any experience where they motivated community residents to improve their health and to become more engaged in their communities.

It was also learned, not surprisingly, that the majority of CHA interventions involved the provision of one-on-one information about diabetes. To better leverage these encounters, the program leaders in NCOMHHD developed a tool that could be used directly with "clients" for the purpose of measuring program effectiveness. This tool allowed for recording of physical activity levels, nutrition matters, and height, weight, and blood pressure of the individuals. This information is meant to be used in two ways: to refer any at-risk individual to appropriate professionals for treatment or to community agencies for other resources. Over a period of 6 months, the CHA will also provide their informal clients with support, nutritional information, and diabetes management tips. The idea was then to readminister the tool and pool results to determine the impact of CHAP intervention. According to key informant Kim Leathers (CHAP Coordinator from the Office of Minority Health & Health Disparities), a university research depart- ·ment is just being engaged to analyse the first set of before-and-after data from the client assessment tool.

Ongoing Training/Support for CHAs

CHAs have regularly identified the need for ongoing training, support, and auxiliary resources. It is recognized that the training components of any lay health education effort are of paramount importance to the success, sustainability, and potential expansion of the program. The NCOMHHD ensures that the various partner organizations, especially the state's community college system, are committed to working with the CHAs. Kim Leathers also pointed out that the occasional confer- ences where the CHAs are brought together are invaluable for training, encouragement, and team-building. Specialized training may become established for team leaders in each church or community organization that has a group of CHAs. Using these secondary leaders more effec- tively for regionalized support and supervision would help the pro- gram to grow while still maintaining quality control. Currently, only two or three supervisors from the NCOMHHD and its Success Dynam- ics contractor try to accomplish all of the oversight. A more fully devel- oped regional organization would bring CHAP more in line with the leadership structure of the CPE program in British Columbia.

There are, in fact, plans to expand CHAP to all 100 counties of North Carolina. Health modules in addition to diabetes will be added to the program via the continuing education courses already provided to CHAs; preventing heart disease and stroke is the new emphasis planned for spring 2010. The training in this area will be available to both new and existing CHAs. As the prevention role of the CHAs be- come more generalized, the long-term vision is that the experience will become a recognized and established career path for community lead- ers seeking a degree in public health or a related field of study.

Case Analysis

Comparisons with British Columbia and the CPE Program

On the face of it, CHAP and the CPE program represent different mod- els. Despite the evident contrasts, CHAP was chosen as a case study for several reasons. First, the focus of CHAP is prevention of chronic disease, with a specific focus on diabetes but with a planned enhancement aimed at including heart disease and stroke. Nutrition and physical activity are two significant components in the toolkit of CHAs, which also overlap with important emphases in the CPE program.

Second, community is the cornerstone of the CHAP program. CHAs are recruited to work with those who are close to them – friends, neighbours, family, church members, etc. – because a trust relationship is already established. This is important for the CHAs because, as non-professionals, they generally prefer to work within their "comfort zone." A close relationship is also important for those receiving the health message, because it is delivered in a familiar and relaxed social setting, and comes from a person they know well. Although CPEs work within a much larger region than a local neighbourhood, having a connection with the community is also a key characteristic of their efforts. Building networks and coalitions while working alongside various community organizations may be seen as a scaled-up version of working with neighbours. This is why the managers of the CPE program give their leaders a head start in this direction by attempting to recruit them from the region where they will be working.

Of course, the preceding discussion also underlines a crucial difference between the two programs. Talking with a neighbour is different from speaking to larger groups and working with coalitions. In fact, CHAP managers are attempting to identify CHAs who might be comfortable speaking at meetings and otherwise mobilizing the community. Committee work and effecting policy change have always been components of CHA training, but most of the ambassadors have not had the experience or aptitude for that level of functioning. The CHAP and CPE programs are essentially about building trust and developing relationships with fellow community members to effectively spread the prevention message – whether at the community level or on a one-to-one basis.

A third reason for selecting CHAP as a case study is precisely because it is a lay health worker model. Lay health workers are not a regular component of the CPE program, but other case studies in this book (e.g., North Karelia, Kentucky) have demonstrated that combining lay health workers and professional leaders in a prevention effort can be very successful. Important lessons may be drawn from CHAP if a lay health worker model is perceived to be a good direction in which to develop a regionalized program.

Insights for the CPE (and Similar) Programs

A dissemination and lay recruitment strategy is potentially important in some remote and/or deprived areas of the province of British Columbia. Recruitment of lay health workers can be extremely challenging. To facilitate the process, CHAP has developed an approach deeply embedded within a network of churches across North Carolina. This strategy has proven to be effective in reaching many different parts of the state, as the church often represents the social backbone of a community. Helpfully, churches and other faith organizations are becoming independently concerned about health disparities. This is a positive development, since they can offer effective channels for delivering health messages to hard-to-reach populations that sometimes distrust the traditional health care system. An equivalent approach could be useful in reaching any minority, underserved, or otherwise vulnerable populations, including those of low socioeconomic status. Adapting this strategy will require creativity in other jurisdictions; it is difficult to reproduce the near-universal community "access" offered by churches in a setting like North Carolina.

Focusing on the motivation of lay health workers is similar to the need to offer support to professional leaders such as CPEs. CHAP managers have recognized the investment required for quality and sustainability of the program. They have placed great emphasis on ensuring that CHAs are fully engaged in the work they are doing, and are motivated to continue over the long term while expanding their knowledge base. Tangible incentives have been added to the program, but the more personal investment represented by attending conferences and workshops is likely of greater importance. Sharing experiences is vital, as is having an opportunity to ask for advice and receive feedback from managers and other mentors.

Conclusion

The lay health worker approach to community-based health interventions is increasingly being applied worldwide for a broad range of health issues. In the state of North Carolina, there is a particular focus on outreach to minority populations such as African Americans. While the focus of CHAP is currently diabetes prevention and control, the lay health worker model can be adapted for any behavioural risk factor prevention, chronic disease management, or other health-related issues.

Lay health workers may be a valuable approach to pursue as the CPE program looks for new avenues to extend its health promotion efforts. However, it may be a model that is most appropriate in ethnocultural groups, including Aboriginal peoples, new Canadians, and other situations where a minority population may exhibit health disparities. However, as useful as lay health workers might be in such settings, it is not clear that the use of churches would be as natural a resource in British Columbia as it is in deprived and/or rural areas of the United States. The opportunities for recruiting and other support may need to be expanded to embrace First Nations bands, other cultural organizations, and other faith-based institutions.

Sources and Further Reading

Campbell MK, Hudson MA, Resnicow K, et al. Church-based health promotion interventions: evidence and lessons learned. Annu Rev Public Health. 2007;28(1):213–34. http://dx.doi.org/10.1146/annurev.publhealth.28.021406.144016. Medline:17155879

North Carolina Diabetes Prevention & Control Fact Sheet. September 2009. Available at http://www.ncdiabetes.org/library/_pdf/DIABETES%20IN%20NC%20WEB.pdf (accessed 28 August 2012).

Plescia M, Groblewski M, Chavis L. A lay health advisor program to promote community capacity and change among change agents. Health Promot Pract. 2008;9(4):434–9. http://dx.doi.org/10.1177/1524839906289670. Medline:17105806

Pullen-Smith B, Carter-Edwards L, Leathers KH. Community health ambassadors: a model for engaging community leaders to promote better health in North Carolina. J Public Health Manag Pract. 2008;(14 Suppl):S73–81. Medline:18843243

9 Manitoba: Health Promotion Coordinators

The health promotion coordinator from the health authority was proud of the First Nations community she had just visited. The local chronic disease prevention committee needed a lot of support, but the members had vision and enthusiasm and were open to her input. The meeting had gone well. She knew the leaders from prevention conferences they had attended with other representatives from around the province. But there was nothing like being on the ground in the community itself. She was especially moved as she walked through the community at the end of the day, heading towards her car and the long drive home. It was the blue lights on the porches of the homes. One by one they came on, adding a blue glow to what seemed like every home. She knew this was the award-winning Blue Light Project, where families wanting to have smoke-free homes signified their commitment with a blue light bulb in their porch socket. The health promotion coordinator knew that this strategy had begun in nine Cree communities in northern Quebec, but now had spread through Manitoba and beyond. She was very involved with its development in this particular community, having helped to secure grant funding and then distributing project materials such as posters, brochures, and … blue light bulbs. As she reached her car, she noticed a front door open and an elder come out; standing on the porch, he lit a cigarette, waved at her, and then pointed up at the blue light bulb and smiled. The health promotion coordinator knew that he felt good about protecting his young children inside, and she also knew that his chances of going all the way and quitting were much higher because of this community-wide effort. That made her smile.

Figure 9.1. Map of Manitoba Regional Health Authorities (RHAs).

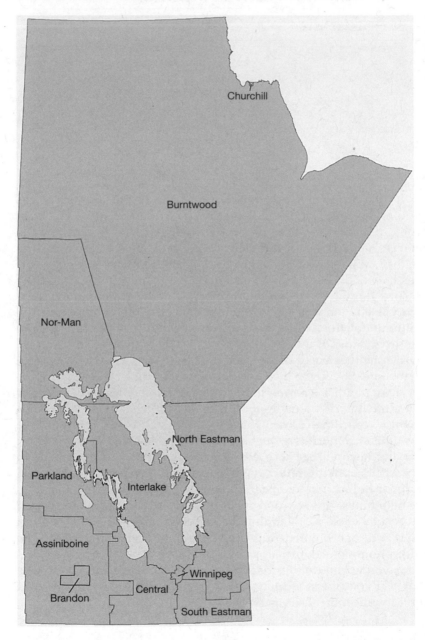

Table 9.1   Manitoba Regional Health Authorities

Regional Health Authority	Population (March 2007)	Size of Health Promotion Team
Winnipeg	667,038	8
Central	101,690	3
Interlake	76,889	5
Assiniboine	68,375	4
South Eastman	61,399	4
Brandon	49,750	6
Burntwood	46,163	2
Parkland	41,725	3
North Eastman	40,157	6
Nor-Man	24,340	5
Churchill	931	2

This case study focuses on the organization and activities of the health promotion staff operating in regional health authorities (RHAs) in the province of Manitoba, Canada.

The current regionalization pattern for health services delivery was established in 1997. There are 11 regional health authorities in Manitoba, with a varying geographical and population base (see Table 9.1). The wide diversity in numbers of people and land area served by each RHA generates unique challenges for regionalization in Manitoba. There are differences between the areas with respect to resources/constraints, organization, and philosophy related to health promotion. However, most of the health authorities do have multiple staff members with job titles incorporating the phrase "health promotion" or a close parallel (e.g., community wellness team). As part of preparing this chapter, several such personnel were contacted from RHAs spanning the province from north to south; they were interviewed in order to better understand the way health promotion has been pursued in Manitoba and to make accurate comparisons with the CPE program in British Columbia. Their thoughtful contributions augmented insights gained from websites and other documentation. One immediate comparison is the fact that the prevention-related staff members have been hired from different fields. There apparently is no single credential or work experience that qualifies a health promotion coordinator to be hired in Manitoba. The background of the interviewees, for example, ranged from recreation/physical activity to public health nursing to anthropology! More standardization may be developing, however. A review has begun of health promotion core competencies (as a subset of public health competencies), identifying key skill sets, etc. Part of the investigation involves building an inventory of position descriptions from across the province.

Health Promotion Activities and Organization

It is clear that one program promoted by Manitoba's Ministry of Health, namely, the Chronic Disease Prevention Initiative (CDPI), has proven to be a watershed for health promotion in the province. Thus, the "modern history" of health promotion strategies and staffing in this Canadian setting may be divided into three phases defined in terms of the CDPI, which was just wrapping up at the time of writing this book:

- Non-CDPI activities (both before and during the initiative)
- Activities related to the active roll-out of the CDPI
- Anticipating the period following the formal CDPI

Activities Outside of the CDPI

A Manitoban perspective on health promotion is suggested in this classic definition adopted by the Burntwood RHA:

> [Health promotion] is the process of enabling people to increase control over and improve their health. This process is based on the understanding that social conditions and personal actions both determine health. Hence, health promotion activities move beyond disease prevention and health education to address social change, institutional change, and community change in addition to changes in personal behaviours.

A further refinement is offered by the role description in the Assiniboine RHA, which stresses the social or community end of the health promotion spectrum:

Our role as health promotion staff is to work with community groups, schools, organizations and public health staff to seek opportunities to improve health.

It is noteworthy that this definition clearly distinguishes health promotion from traditional public health roles.

The health promotion workers in Manitoba's RHAs have been innovative in developing community-based interventions for health change, many of which predate the CDPI. There is an acknowledged commitment to developing programs in an evidence-based manner as much as possible. Leaders in Manitoba are aided in fulfilling this standard by consulting reviews of evidence. In fact, the volume of review activity has necessitated the invention of a new level of information synthesis, dubbed the "review of reviews." An example of the latter type of project in a Canadian context is the Knowledge Exchange Network (KEN), sponsored by the Canadian Cancer Society – Manitoba Division. Motivated by information found in KEN and other sources, RHAs in Manitoba have been involved with the following types of initiatives:

- Purchasing exercise treadmills for the public and clients of health agencies in the town of Thompson, as well as for outlying communities in the widespread Burntwood RHA
- Sponsoring community walking events
- Providing a bus to facilitate low-income children taking advantage of a winter recreational park
- Healthy breakfast programs in schools and large, colourful "What's in Your Lunch?" information posters
- Physical activity leadership development program involving new sports coaches, swimming instructors, etc.
- Community gardens and other food security initiatives
- New strategies for male health, especially related to workplace programs

Encouraging personal change through standard forms of health education has also been pursued through Manitoba RHAs; closely related to this is biological risk factor screening, which can spur behaviour change. For instance, the health promotion team in one RHA administers a project fund, offering grants of up to $1,000 for community projects aimed at healthy eating, physical activity, smoking cessation, and stress reduction. As will be described below, this "community grant" approach is similar to one of the pillars of the CDPI. Other health education platforms in Manitoba can be found in many parts of Canada, including mobile wellness events that occur at workplaces, community fairs, First Nation treaty days, etc. These events are designed to provide education on the common risk factors of chronic disease and offer a foundation for clinical prevention among at-risk individuals through blood pressure and blood sugar checks and BMI measurements.

In addition, there are signs of health promotion strategies being pushed beyond community programs and individual behaviour change to broader environmental/policy matters. For instance, the Assiniboine RHA has advocated healthy food choices in recreation facilities and the reinforcement of smoke-free spaces. The effort has been formalized under the heading "Making the Move to Healthy Choices." The program has been picked up by New Brunswick and Quebec, with Hamilton, Ontario, also expressing interest.

Finally, secondary prevention sometimes appears to be a priority under the health promotion umbrella in Manitoba, although it is arguable that this represents an awkward fit with a classic health promotion perspective. The secondary prevention efforts found in several Manitoba RHAs focus on screening and self-management programs related to chronic diseases such as diabetes.

Organization Predating CDPI

The differences between RHAs in terms of health promotion organization and philosophy were noted earlier. It is of interest that about a third of the RHAs have chosen to explicitly integrate health promotion into a broader theme of "primary health care." This is a conceptual framework first introduced at a 1978 World Health Organization conference held in Alma Ata, Kazakhstan (then part of the USSR). Inspired by federal-provincial strategizing and federal funding commitments, a plan to guide the development of a primary health care approach within Manitoba was approved in April 2002. Despite the confusing similarity in terminology, primary health care is not the same thing as primary care (i.e., "the medical care received on first contact with the medical system, before being referred elsewhere"). The definition of primary health care incorporates the philosophy of accessing clinical and public health care where one lives, works, and plays. Further, a commitment to primary health care calls for the most appropriate health care to be delivered by the most appropriate provider and methods in the most appropriate setting. Community-based, multidisciplinary teams have emerged globally as a cornerstone strategy to accomplish this pattern of health care. More pertinent to the topic of this book, primary health care is intended to influence arenas beyond the health sector when it addresses the broader social determinants of health, and to create and build on a foundation of community participation.

Reflecting the community orientation at the heart of the definition, primary health care activity has been divided geographically in some health authorities in Manitoba. For example, the North Eastman RHA has five health planning districts, each with a Primary Health Care Centre staffed by an interdisciplinary team of health professionals. There appears to be a "team within a team" that specifically focuses on chronic disease prevention and management. Each of these specialized teams comprises at least the following staff members:

- Primary health care nurses focusing on individual and community education about healthy lifestyles
- Clinical/community dieticians
- Wellness facilitators who, among other duties, take responsibility for the needs assessment, community engagement, and intersectoral mobilization aspects of health promotion

This sort of district-level reproduction of a relatively comprehensive prevention team may be contrasted with other RHAs where the geographical distribution of staff is less uniform. However, the latter sort of pattern, as illustrated by the Assiniboine RHA (see Figure 9.2), still has the advantage of avoiding a concentration of all resources in one central town in the health authority.

Activities Related to CDPI

The design of the Chronic Disease Prevention Initiative (CDPI) was influenced by previous prevention activity in the province, especially the Manitoba Heart Health Project. The latter was the Manitoba arm of the Canadian Heart Health Initiative (CHHI), a countrywide strategy for the prevention of cardiovascular disease that ran from 1986 to 2006. The CHHI entailed an extensive coalition involving Health Canada, the 10 provincial departments of health, and over 1,000 other organizations.

Figure 9.2. Map of Assiniboine RHA.

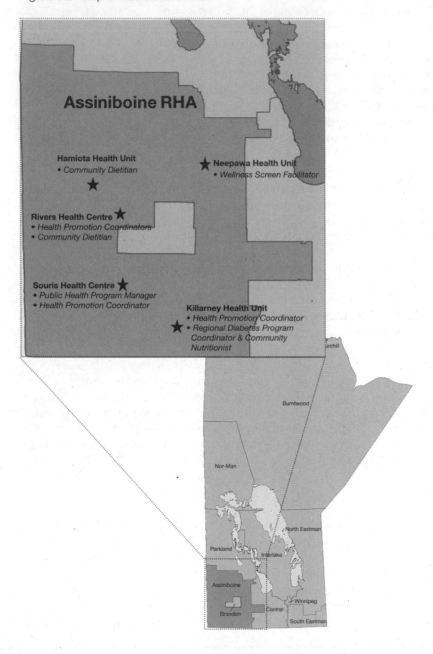

There were five phases: policy development through countrywide consultations (1986–88); provincial heart health surveys (1986–91); research demonstration programs within provinces (1989–97); evaluation (1994–97); and an extended dissemination research period allowing for studies of the sustained adoption of interventions by communities and health systems. Ultimately, several elements of the CHHI informed the development of the CDPI. The CDPI was the product of a multisectoral planning process to address the primary prevention of not just heart disease but chronic disease more broadly. Direction was received through an advisory committee of key decision-makers drawn from the federal and provincial governments, non-governmental organizations, and RHAs; the committee initiated and guided a 2-year consultative process to design the initiative.

The CDPI was constructed as a 5-year community-focused plan (2005–10) employing a comprehensive, integrated approach that emphasized local partnerships, citizen engagement, and community development in order to reduce the incidence of premature morbidity and mortality related to chronic disease in Manitoba. CancerCare Manitoba has had a shared leadership role in risk factor surveillance, monitoring, and evaluation efforts. The conditions of interest included cancer, cardiovascular disease, diabetes, kidney disease, and lung disease, plus the three classic modifiable risk factors common to most of those conditions: smoking, physical inactivity, and unhealthy eating.

Consensus was achieved concerning the following objectives and approaches:

- Fostering public involvement and local actions
- Using evidence-based decision-making
- Increasing upstream investment to help create supportive environments that make an individual's choice for health the easiest choice
- Applying multiple strategies by collaborating horizontally and vertically with all sectors and levels of society
- Addressing the social determinants of health and their interactions
- Utilizing a population-based health approach
- Supporting community capacity development with commitment to reducing health disparities

Substantial aspects of the implementation of CDPI depended on the regional health authorities. The connection with RHAs involved two critical components of CDPI: grants to selected "high risk" communities to mount locally adapted risk factor prevention activities; and provincial and regional support and accountability. The grant typically amounted to $2 per community member per year; stringent standards had to be met in order to qualify. Helping community leaders to manage the application and evaluation processes was a typical assignment for health promotion officers in Manitoba. Indeed, the time involvement of RHA staff members during the life of the CDPI was quite high, complementing the commitment of community organizers. For instance, the Burntwood RHA in the north of Manitoba had 22 communities involved with the granting process. This involved time investment by local leaders, a functioning advisory committee, and relatively demanding processes of reporting.

There was variation in how each RHA in the province handled its support role with the communities involved. The Burntwood RHA had to be creative, given its large pool of communities eligible for the CDPI – especially since the majority of the areas had no resident RHA staff and were only accessible by air (or, in some cases, by ice road in the winter). In fact, a large proportion of the 22 communities were First Nations reserves where health care is by law a federal responsibility and thus there was little track record of RHA involvement. Ultimately, the geographical, workload, and other barriers were overcome by convening a conference in Thompson where the community leaders could come to complete their CDPI application, receive information and training, and be paired with a staff member from the RHA who would act as a part-time liaison and support person over the years of the initiative. The actual health promotion coordinator, rather than being overwhelmed by so many communities and community projects, was able to provide oversight and act as a convenor and morale booster for a team.

Activities in the Post-CDPI Era

The post-CDPI period in Manitoba has really just begun. RHAs will be challenged from a budgetary perspective to maintain the momentum generated by CDPI, especially its granting mechanism and resources. Unless sufficient local capacity-building was accomplished before the end of the CDPI and/or grants are generated from some other source, there is the real possibility that the various community-based projects in the province will come to an end at some point. Fortunately, the province is continuing to flow funding to the regions in the current transitional year. Although the amounts are reduced (with some partner funding ending as of 31 March 2010), certain community action plans could be sustained through 2011–12. Beyond this, some new resources have been put in place to keep the momentum going. This time Manitoba Health and Healthy Living has decided to fund core staffing to expand health promotion and related staffing within the RHAs. The aim is to allow regions to strengthen an integrated team approach to chronic disease prevention and healthy living across the province – hence the name of the expanded staff complement: Healthy Living Teams. Of course, funding for core personnel has been very welcome, but it remains to be seen how the new staff resources will be deployed to maintain the benefits generated by CDPI in multiple communities throughout the province. Finally, while CDPI developed certain aspects of the evaluation capacity, key informants from the RHAs consistently noted that much more needed to happen in terms of tracking intermediate and ultimate outcomes and adding to the evidence base concerning effectiveness of interventions.

Case Analysis

The same approach will be applied as in the other case studies, first looking for comparisons between the context and content of the programs in British Columbia and Manitoba, and then drawing out insights that are relevant to a CPE-like approach to cancer and other chronic disease prevention.

Comparisons with British Columbia and the CPE Program

GEOPOLITICAL SETTING
British Columbia and Manitoba are both Canadian provinces, so there are of course many overlaps, including the dominance of the provincial government in health care planning and delivery. Both jurisdictions have chosen to mete out health care services through regional health authorities. Manitoba has twice the number of RHAs serving a quarter of British Columbia's population. As in British Columbia, the citizens are spread across a vast landscape, stretching from more densely populated centres in the south (and therefore near the U.S. border) to small, remote communities in the north. The Winnipeg Regional Health Authority is the only RHA that approximates the complexity of the urban health authorities in British Columbia's "Lower Mainland."

Both provinces have a substantial Aboriginal population living both on and off reserves. British Columbia has the second-largest such population in Canada (after Ontario) in absolute terms, but the *proportion* of the Manitoba population that is Aboriginal is higher. There are 63 First Nations communities in Manitoba, many in isolated northern settings. Both provinces deal with jurisdictional issues, since the federal government has formal responsibility for health care on reserves. The Manitoba Aboriginal groupings are more varied; about a third of Aboriginal peoples in the province are Métis, and there are a small number of Inuit.

British Columbia and Manitoba both have a long history of immigration, although it is fair to say that the recent influx in British Columbia has been more intensive and has involved more visible minorities. As western provinces, both jurisdictions have a strong tradition of agriculture and industries based on natural resource extraction; the contemporary economy of British Columbia is now more diversified.

FOCUS AND APPROACH

Both the CPE program in British Columbia and the RHA-based health promotion activities in Manitoba generally address the classic risk factors of chronic disease, with the following notable features:

- The British Columbia program of course has a cancer prevention focus and therefore also deals with cancer-specific risk factors such as excessive ultraviolet radiation exposure
- Similarly, supporting cancer secondary prevention (i.e., screening) is an additional focus of the CPE program
- Health promotion staff in Manitoba have tended to address the risk factor of stress alongside the traditional categories of tobacco use, nutrition, and physical activity

CPEs in British Columbia and the comparable officers in Manitoba are equally committed to a health promotion perspective in accomplishing their task. This means embracing strategies beyond service delivery per se; in particular, health promotion is understood to be bigger than health education, as traditionally defined. Importantly, community engagement approaches represent a consistent commitment within both the British Columbia and Manitoba programs.

TEAM CHARACTERISTICS

As introduced in chapter 4, there are good parallels between the health promotion staff in Manitoba and the four dimensions abstracted from the CPE model. In addition to an overlap around the community engagement strategy, the Manitoba RHA personnel are professionals (and employed full-time in their role, in contrast with the CPEs); furthermore, they bring a mostly generalist prevention perspective to bear on a defined population. As with most CPEs, the target populations in Manitoba are defined geographically. In the case of the North Eastman RHA, the areas of coverage are sub-regional. Such formal subdivision is the exception, although attempts have been made to distribute the staff geographically in other RHAs. As described above, managing the CDPI-funded projects sometimes called for staff resources to be temporarily spread around a region in terms of assignment, if not in terms of location of residence.

Whether they were distributed within a region or not, the main contrast with the situation in British Columbia is that every Manitoba RHA has a *team* of staff members working on health promotion and chronic disease matters. This maximizes the opportunity for collegial support, sharing interests and skill sets, etc., especially when compared with the solo CPEs who sometimes cover large areas and/or large populations. There is about a 1:200,000 staff-to-population ratio in British Columbia (lower if the part-time status of the workers is considered), but the Manitoba ratio is more like 1:20,000, different by an order of magnitude. Of course, as described below, the CPEs do not represent the entirety of health promotion leadership in the various areas of British Columbia.

Another pertinent organizational difference involves the fact that CPEs occupy a unique quasi-governmental role compared to the less equivocal *official* status enjoyed by RHA staff. A theme that emerges in other case studies in this book is that community organizers can sometimes take advantage of a perceived unofficial status, one which sometimes creates greater openness to health promotion overtures among individuals and community groups, and greater possibilities to enter into partnerships with unorthodox allies such as businesses. In short, there is sometimes resistance to government agents "telling us what to do." On the other hand, such resistance may be overcome by dedication to community engagement principles and practices.

As a tangential note, there are in fact other, more overtly official health promotion leaders in British Columbia, including staff committed to this purpose within each RHA. Interestingly, a scan of the health authority websites in British Columbia reveals that, unlike in Manitoba, the health promotion activities are mediated through staff members whose job title explicitly includes "health promotion." A description of such work, whatever its label, is offered by the Interior Health Authority in British Columbia:

> The Healthy Community Environment program uses an integrated approach to improve human health by creating a healthier built environment. A variety of Interior Health employees will work collaboratively to encourage people to lead healthy lives and promote community planning and design which prevents potential environmental and social threats. The components of the Healthy Community Environment program consist of community responsiveness, collaboration for healthy community environments, and research and program evaluation.

Certain health authorities in British Columbia make it clear that public health nurses, usually working out of local health units, are the lead staff members in at least some of these matters. Finally, a commitment to the primary health care model is central to the delivery of health promotion in some of the health authorities, matching the approach seen in parts of Manitoba. The spectrum of "official" prevention services, strategies, and workers within the health authorities of British Columbia underlines one arena of partnership that should be pursued by CPEs in fulfilling their collaboration mandate.

Insights for the CPE (and Similar) Programs

A number of factors may be identified as influences on successful, or at least promising, chronic disease prevention efforts in Manitoba. These insights can also reinforce or inform the ongoing commitments and strategies of CPEs in British Columbia.

First, it seems that more intensive staffing may lead to better results. After recent funding for additional healthy living staff, the ratio of health promotion coordinators (or their equivalents) to population has been improved to about 1:20,000.

Second, a strategic way to develop coordinator capacity is to aim for (and fund) sub-regional coverage. This model is consistent with the district-level staffing seen in some parts of Manitoba. The parallel unit for CPEs to cover in the British Columbia context may be some new aggregation of local health areas that would improve the average staff-to-population ratio from the current 1:200,000. The recent multiplication of staff in Manitoba continues to underline the importance of drawing prevention/health promotion staff from the region or district being served. To paraphrase an RHA worker in one Manitoba community: "I grew up in this town, and my own family is growing up here now. It is important to know the local needs in order to represent them well. I am extra motivated because, for instance, my daughter will benefit from improved sports facilities and coaching. I know a lot of people, making it easier to create and maintain connections on community coalitions. We have more than a theoretical interest; we have a vested interest."

Next, even when a helpful sense of "team" is created across multiple health promotion coordinators in a region, the assignment still calls more for generalists than specialists. That is why there has been a natural evolution in Manitoba from, for instance, being a tobacco control specialist to being a true health promotion coordinator. To build further on this pattern, coordinators are being exposed to training in emerging arenas such as physical activity interventions. Similarly, diabetes management workers are transitioning to roles where they deal with chronic disease in general. Ultimately, communities need to be equipped to address all of the critical risk factors; this comprehensive perspective should inform the central role of a community-based cancer (or chronic disease) prevention educator.

Finally, benefits may be eroded when experiencing a pendulum swing between community projects and core operations staffing. This sort of shift has marked Manitoba as it transitions to the post-CDPI era. Funding is really needed in *both* arenas to generate an advance in terms of community development that can be well supported by health promotion professionals. As one key informant in Manitoba noted, it is difficult to *get* community partners to the table and to *get* some planning energy from them when there is nothing tangible to *give* them to make their efforts more productive. Further, as noted by CDPI Training Coordinator Betty Kozak, many communities and regions were able to garner additional funding from partners by leveraging what they were now able to "bring to the table" through CDPI funding, rather than always presenting themselves as the "poor cousins." Optimally, funding professional support staff and funding community-inspired projects should go hand-in-hand.

Conclusion

This case study has been built around understanding the "before, during, and after" of the Chronic Disease Prevention Initiative in Manitoba. It was an important program. The CDPI has been a catalyst for developments that are very consistent with a health promotion approach to chronic disease prevention. Notably, its key strategy of community grants is closely tied to the health promotion perspective, specifically in terms of local needs assessment, local planning, and local buy-in. Among other benefits, the community focus inspired by the CDPI generated a further practical subdivision of some regions; the mobilization of local efforts was reminiscent of the permanent districts and dispersed primary health care teams found in an RHA such as North Eastman. The main difference is that the CDPI community-based work generally did not entail on-site core staffing and other permanent resources. Nonetheless, the value generated within RHAs during the life of the CDPI is undeniable: prevention projects tailored to local needs were of direct benefit to community members, many (albeit part-time) health promotion supporters were mobilized with a specific geographical focus, robust training was received by community leaders and RHA support staff through Manitoba Health events, and there was new access to First Nations communities that had typically been very isolated. This underlines the potential catalytic value of funds being available for community projects and community capacity-building. It is therefore a program element that could enhance the effectiveness of CPEs in British Columbia, especially in under-resourced regions and communities.

  Sustainability, however, will always be an issue. Manitoba and British Columbia would both benefit from a consistent stream of funding for building local leadership capacity and maintaining chronic disease prevention programs tailored to local populations. The unique contribution of community-based prevention coordinators also needs to be protected. Conversations with health promotion staff in Manitoba underlined just how fragile their role can be. First, health promotion, especially its central community development role, is often not very well understood, and this means that any orphan public health function can end up being parked under its umbrella. Moreover, the activity of chronic disease prevention needs to be well integrated with other core health care functions, and then well evaluated in terms of effectiveness in reducing risky behaviours and improving health status, lest it become the first program that is cut when funds become tight.

Sources and Further Reading

Canadian Cancer Society – Manitoba Division. Knowledge Exchange Network. Available at http://www.cancer.ca/Manitoba/Prevention/MB-Knowledge%20Exchange%20Network.aspx (accessed 8 January 2010).

CDPI Funding News Release. 2011. Available at http://news.gov.mb.ca/news/index.html?archive=&item=10760 (accessed July 2011).

Chronic Disease Prevention Initiative. An Evaluation of the Chronic Disease Prevention Initiative (CDPI) Executive Summary. 2010. Available at http://www.healthincommon.ca/wp-content/uploads/Evaluation-Executive-Summary.pdf (accessed 3 March 2010).

Chronic Disease Prevention Initiative – Project Charter. Available at http://www.healthincommon.ca/ (accessed July 2011).

Health Council of Canada. Primary health care teams – a Manitoba perspective. Available at http://www.healthcouncilcanada.ca/ (accessed July 2011).

Robinson K, Farmer T, Elliott SJ, et al. From heart health promotion to chronic disease prevention: contributions of the Canadian Heart Health Initiative. Prev Chronic Dis. 2007;4(2):A29. Medline:17362620

PART C

A Strategic Pattern for Prevention Educators

10 Important Elements of a CPE-like Program

As stated in the introductory chapter, the ultimate purpose of this book is to provide an evidence base and template for planners considering a strategy similar to the Community-Based Prevention Educator (CPE) program in British Columbia. To serve this end, this chapter will identify important elements that should be considered when building such a program.

What is the argument for including the elements described in this chapter? In each instance, the element or characteristic fulfils one or more of the following criteria:

- A feature that is common to two or more programs examined
- An area needing improvement that is highlighted by two or more programs
- A substantial component found in a sustained and/or successful program such as the North Karelia Project

On this basis, nine areas emerged that can be characterized as important. Before turning to a brief overview of each such element, an explanation is warranted. The reader will note that the following four points are *not* included in the list: the prevention educators should be professionals, they should be regionally deployed or otherwise have a clearly delineated target population, they should concentrate on community engagement, and the prevention agenda ought to be of a generalist nature. These key points are not included because they constitute the definitional grid that informed the case study selection. In other words, all the prevention educator programs considered in the book reflect these four features *by definition*. To include them here as some form of inductively discovered elements would be superfluous.

The nine "success factors" that legitimately emerge from the analysis comprise the following:

1 Using educators who have familiarity with the region and who can build on existing relationships
2 An intensive staff-to-population ratio
3 Pilot projects that are scalable (i.e., have the potential for expansion)
4 Comprehensive risk factor targets and societal settings
5 Primary *and* secondary prevention focus
6 Strong university affiliation
7 Using lay health advisers or other types of volunteer educators
8 Media messages to reinforce the other work, consistent across partner organizations
9 Enhancements (such as mobile prevention units) to increase access to services

After a presentation to the CPEs who reviewed this inventory, it was encouraging that follow-up interviews confirmed the validity of the list. Each of the "success factors" will be outlined in the sections below.

Local Knowledge and Connections to the Region

Intrinsic to any CPE-like role is a deep-rooted connection to the communities in which the CPE works. Many of British Columbia's CPEs were either raised in the regions they serve or have spent years living in the area. This is also the case for several of the health promotion coordinators in Manitoba. Some commented on the personal investment in their communities that is inspired by their own young families as well as past generations of family members. There is extra motivation when the health of one's own family is invested in the project. Beyond motivational factors, it is not surprising that building networks, developing collaborations, and mobilizing the community are facilitated by having long-standing relationships with local leaders and citizens. A further advantage to health promotion staff having roots in their communities is that they are more likely to be committed to the position over the long term. A high quality, sustained effort is vital to the success of many programs; staff turnover is naturally detrimental to building community relationships, especially in cultures where personal trust is a key lubricant for moving plans forward. Finally, deep community roots tap into a wellspring of community pride. There is power when "we" are engaged to achieve collective success. Given these forces, it is unsurprising that an effective program such as the North Karelia Project boasted staff and supporters who had been in place for decades. Likewise, the Kentucky Cancer Program has had some cancer control specialists on assignment in their regions for well over 10 years.

Ratio of Prevention Educators to Population

One of the quantitative metrics that can be drawn from the CPE program in British Columbia and the highlighted case studies is the ratio of workers to the population that they serve (see Table 10.1 below). The implication of a smaller ratio is straightforward: greater staff resources within a jurisdiction, and thus smaller target populations, will enable more intensive prevention activities.

The Health Education through Extension Leadership (HEEL) program in Kentucky, with an average of 1 staff member for every 6,000 individuals in the population, appears to be an outlier. As noted in the case study of this program, one key informant confirmed that such intensive staffing is a result of a pattern established decades ago and suggested that replicating the approach would be unfeasible in today's economic climate. Beyond this anomaly, there appear to be two distinct orders of magnitude among the other programs. The first category falls in the 1:20,000 to 1:30,000 range, where the other is about 10 times less intense in terms of staffing, between 1:200,000 and 1:300,000. It appears that programs with a strict focus on cancer (e.g., Action Cancer in Northern Ireland, the Kentucky Cancer Program) have a lower staffing ratio than those with a broader chronic disease prevention agenda (e.g., the North Karelia Project or the Manitoba Regional Health Authorities). In theoretical terms, this may be explicable in terms of the higher strategic demands created by the broader agenda. More practically, staffing complements come down to budgets. The planners and advocates involved with chronic diseases may have a tendency to raise or invest more funds in prevention. Cancer-specific programs could benefit from stressing the overlap of risk factors and the potential for reducing several diseases through the efforts of a CPE-like program.

British Columbia, at 1:200,000, falls into the second category; in fact, taking into consideration that the CPEs in that province only work part-time, the ratio ought to be pegged even lower. Based on international

Table 10.1 Staff-to-Population Ratio of Relevant Community Health Promotion Programs

Position Title (Program Name)	Jurisdiction	Staff : Population Ratio
Field Office Staff Team (North Karelia Project)	Finland	1 : 30,000
Health Promotion Officers (Action Cancer)	Northern Ireland	1 : 300,000
Cancer Control Specialists (Kentucky Cancer Program)	Kentucky	1 : 300,000
Extension Agents (Health Education through Extension Leadership)	Kentucky	1 : 6,000
Community-Based Prevention Educators (CPE Program)	British Columbia	1 : 200,000
Health Promotion Coordinators (Regional Health Authorities)	Manitoba	1 : 20,000

models, this suggests that there is good reason to expand the CPE team in British Columbia.

Pilot Approach Followed by Program Expansion (Scalability)

Expansion of a program to new regions or population groups is usually an indicator of its success. Several of the case studies discussed in this book have spread beyond the original area targeted by CPE-like efforts. For instance, the prevention activity in the province of North Karelia was a demonstration project, intended from the outset to be a pilot for all of Finland (as well as being carefully monitored from the beginning in terms of its global implications). After the manifest early success of the program, it was expanded to the entire country within 5 years. The British Columbia CPE program also had its beginnings as a pilot program – known as the Waddell Project – before growing into a province-wide initiative.

There are a number of advantages to demonstrating a project on a limited scale before committing to nationwide implementation. The feasibility of the project may be assessed, including the identification of logistical problems, resource requirements, staff training needs, etc. Most critically, the health effects, other outcomes, and general experience of the project may be evaluated. Proven success on a regional level also brings a project into focus for key stakeholders – including government, other potential funding organizations, and the general public. This creates the all-important momentum and "buy-in" that will hopefully lead to a commitment of resources to expand a project and ensure that it can be sustained.

Some programs are not officially characterized as pilot projects in the beginning, but they may still become models on which expanded programs are based. For example, the Community Health Ambassador Program (CHAP) in North Carolina was established as a diabetes prevention initiative, since that chronic disease represents one of the biggest health issues there. Although it began in only a small proportion of the state's counties, it has spread to more areas, and there are now plans to expand to all 100 counties. In addition, there are plans to expand the CHAP mandate to include other chronic diseases such as heart disease and stroke.

Finally, it is important to note that investigators and theorists are very interested in the pattern of spread of new programs and the forces at work. There can be a combination of intentional mechanisms (planned dissemination and adaptation) and more spontaneous adoption of new ideas and approaches. The latter is closely connected with an influential theory known as diffusion of innovations, a topic that will be explored further in the next chapter.

Comprehensive Targets and Platforms

The North Karelia Project resulted in significant positive changes in health behaviours. One reason for its success was a commitment to a comprehensive prevention approach. The project comprised a multi-component initiative that was implemented at multiple levels in society – individual, community, institutional, and public policy – and in a variety of settings, from primary care to schools to workplaces. Such extensive and intensive intervention approaches represent the sort of evidence-based strategy recommended for effecting health behaviour changes across a population. There are many terms that describe a commitment to move beyond clinical or educational strategies that only focus on changing individual behaviours; a common name for this approach is the "socioecologic model." Writing for the Centers for Disease Control, specifically regarding North Carolina, Plescia and colleagues stated that "a socioecologic approach to community health recognizes that health behaviors are multifaceted and are part of a larger social system of behaviors and social influences." This is why the full health promotion efforts in that state are designed to encompass more than the one-to-one work of the Community Health Ambassador Program (CHAP); it also explains why CHAP is committed to recruiting lay health workers who are more qualified to speak about the social determinants of health.

Although the socioecologic arena is recognized as critical to supporting behavioural change in individuals and groups, implementing policy and other environmental change is a difficult process. Most of the stories of prevention educators effecting such change relate to neighbourhoods or perhaps the municipal or regional health authority level; influencing higher levels of government, industry, and the health care system typically require the involvement of more senior prevention leaders and planners working in parallel with the regional efforts of a prevention educator. Whatever the societal level at stake, most of the prevention educator models examined for this book involve government funding; this means that there are traditional limitations on direct advocacy work. Intriguingly, the one model that involved private funding – the Action Cancer charity in Northern Ireland – does not include advocacy as part of the health promotion officer assignment. In British Columbia, it seems that some degree of policy focus is expected, as seen in the following line from the CPE job description: "Assist management by coordinating regional field work of province wide action initiatives e.g., letter-writing campaigns." Even in this case, however, it seems that CPEs tend to work indirectly as policy change agents, supplying evidence and other information to committees and coalitions in order to shape their joint advocacy campaigns.

One platform for prevention intervention that is sometimes neglected is primary care. This gap has been explicitly acknowledged in the British Columbia Cancer Agency Prevention Programs, and identified as a quality improvement priority. Primary care providers could be a fruitful target of in-service training in the area of prevention, but it is not clear if community-based prevention educators have the time or expertise to exploit this opportunity. As seen in initiatives such as the North Karelia Project, motivated primary care partners would have much to offer in terms of advocacy, service delivery, referrals, etc. in the advancement of the cause of chronic disease prevention.

Beyond Primary Prevention

Although primary prevention often is the main focus of a chronic disease prevention program, secondary prevention activities – mostly involving screening – can be integrated into such programs to great effect. The CPEs in British Columbia have generally had a very positive experience with increased attention to screening education and promotion. They have found that screening initiatives have frequently offered an entrée, leading to primary prevention opportunities. Screening is an important aspect of both the Kentucky Cancer Program and Action Cancer in Northern Ireland. A version of screening was also an early part of the North Karelia Project; rather than identifying disease precursors per se, the focus was on a biological precursor, specifically hypertension. Importantly, screening campaigns can integrate two other success factors noted later in this chapter, namely, the use of media/marketing and the deployment of "accessibility tools" such as mobile screening units.

Besides screening, another type of advanced prevention comprises disease management that is aimed at avoiding complications. For example, a growing part of North Carolina's CHAP mandate is to provide diabetes self-management education that is designed to avoid the well-known complications of diabetes.

Finally, tertiary prevention is also emerging as a target of CPE activities in British Columbia, specifically with respect to reducing the incidence of second primary cancers in cancer survivors. Among other practitioners, Italian oncologists Veronesi and Bonani recently stressed the importance of tertiary prevention efforts aimed at second primary cancers. The latter malignancies represent no small matter: as a class, the cases of a new cancer following an experience of a first cancer are the sixth most frequent type of cancer encountered in the world.

University Research Partnerships

Three of the case studies examined in this book – Kentucky HEEL, Kentucky Cancer Program, and the North Karelia Project – demonstrate strong affiliations with universities. In each instance, this aspect of the program was cited as a key to its success. The majority of the literature in this area relates to a specific paradigm, community-based participatory research (CBPR). There are a number of close synonyms used for the approach, including action research, translational research, and community health partnerships. It constitutes a relatively new methodology, with a quarter of the papers with an explicit reference to CBPR being published in the last 6 months. In 1998, Israel and colleagues described CBPR as follows: "A collaborative approach to research that equitably involves, for example, community members, organizational representatives, and researchers in all aspects of the research process. The partners contribute unique strengths and shared responsibilities to enhance understanding of a given phenomenon and the social and cultural dynamics of the community, and integrate the knowledge gained with action to improve the health and well-being of community members."

Connecting communities to researchers extends well beyond one method or philosophy, but the principles related to CBPR are still instructive. The practice of CBPR confirms that partnerships forged between community-based prevention educators and academic researchers can provide multiple benefits, including:

- Consideration of conceptual frameworks (as developed in academic settings) in the overall planning of the educator strategy
- Trust-building between researchers and community members who are a target of research interest, allowing for more liberal access to community-based data
- Engendering a consistent "culture of learning," including the critical importance of evaluation in the planning-implementation-improvement cycle
- Guidance on evaluation protocols around prevention efforts, from data collection to analysis to reporting
- Incorporating local knowledge and energy into the design and implementation of research programs and projects
- Fostering community action as part of a research project, or as a result of research outcomes, with a good promise of positive effects for community members
- Generating and distributing resources to fund projects that may in turn help a community, for example, a small grants program
- Developing reports and articles for publication, which can be a source of pride and motivation for community members and organizers alike

What becomes clear in the preceding list is that community-based research efforts have the potential to produce reciprocal benefits, where the agenda of investigators/organizers and the needs of community members are both fulfilled. There is also mutuality in the information exchanged. University faculty members and students bring knowledge of research literature and methods that point towards best practices, including novel technologies; community members and prevention educators bring past experience with interventions, as well as knowledge of the region and its population and cultural and other contextual characteristics. Acknowledging the resources in both realms, and drawing appropriate lessons from them, creates a foundation for reciprocal learning and results in relationships built on trust and respect, as well as a sense of empowerment – especially for community members.

Most of the principles described above are amply demonstrated in the story of the North Karelia Project in Finland. Although British Columbia's prevention educators were founded with solid theoretical input from the academic world (see the next chapter), the connection seems to be less developed in the current structure of the CPE program. The potential value of academic collaboration may be especially high given the international reputation of the parent organization – the British Columbia Cancer Agency – as a research institution, and the presence of so many world-class universities in the province. That said, the BCCA PEL program was developed to implement that which is proven.

Volunteer Educators (Such as Lay Health Advisers)

Lay health advisers are "natural helpers" in the community who advise and assist their neighbours with a variety of health issues. As described by Nemcek and Sabatier: "They possess indigenous qualities of the subculture such as verbal and nonverbal language skills; racial/ethnic qualities of the subculture; social/environmental familiarity; and an understanding of the community's health beliefs, health behaviours, and barriers to health services." "Lay" in the title of this role refers to various ways in which it is a "non-professional" assignment, including not having a formal health credential and not being paid. As outlined in chapter 4, these features generally set the role apart from a job such as community-based prevention educators. There are many alternate terms used for lay health advisers, including community health ambassadors (as in CHAP in North Carolina), peer educators, community health workers, and community health promoters (translated as *promotoras de salud* in Hispanic contexts in the United States). It is a model that has become increasingly popular around the world.

As noted by Chronic Disease Director Marcus Plescia in North Carolina, lay health advisers "enhance empowerment and capacity building by promoting and supporting individuals who assume responsibility for community improvement, seek new knowledge and skills, and actively engage and recruit others." A special type of recruiting facilitated by lay health advisers involves populating community-based participatory research projects (see the previous section), although care must be taken around certain ethical issues that arise in such contexts. Closely allied with a more systematic coverage of neighbourhoods with lay health advisers is the employment of opinion leaders, such as community elders, to influence the attitudes of whole communities in a more diffuse manner.

The lay health adviser or opinion leader models can be effective as a discrete program, but this does not need to be a stand-alone effort. The case studies focusing on North Karelia and Kentucky (both the HEEL and Kentucky Cancer Programs) illustrated that lay health leaders can be highly effective when combined with professional health promotion staff. The integration of lay health advisers with British Columbia's CPE program may be of particular value in reaching immigrant populations and more remote areas of the province, including certain Aboriginal communities.

Media and Marketing Efforts with Accurate and Consistent Messages

Most comprehensive community-based prevention programs employ some media and marketing as part of the effort. The strategic questions related to this approach are as follows: how much focus should there be on media messaging, who should be in charge of maintaining a consistent message, where are resources best invested to maximize effectiveness, and what opportunities are there for "free" publicity?

The most robust example of media coverage from the case studies was once again provided by the model program in North Karelia, where television, radio, and print sources were used extensively to promote the prevention initiatives. One of the best known examples was an early version of reality television, where the participants were selected from the pool of citizens trying to reduce their risk factors.

The informants from each model program agreed on the importance of media messaging to complement other efforts. In addition to direct impacts on an audience, media campaigns can generate the additional benefit of legitimizing the regular work of prevention educators; there can be a crossover effect in this regard, where, for instance, a screening campaign can lead to client contacts that can be leveraged for the sake of other behavioural interventions. Given the potential effects of high-quality marketing, program leaders generally acknowledged that formulating and disseminating information in a creative manner is a complex task that requires expert input from the central program office or a consultant.

Action Cancer, the service charity in Northern Ireland, represents a strong example of how creative advertising and marketing can create awareness of a program's goals and objectives. It also demonstrates how funding may be obtained through corporate sponsorships if the circumstances are favourable; examples include the Big Bus subsidy provided by Super Valu-Centra and the "Smokers Face" campaign supported by Gordon's Chemists. Of course, this sort of private sponsorship is generally not as acceptable in publicly managed programs.

One of the most persistent problems facing prevention programs today is competition from unhelpful or untrue information. Project leaders from North Karelia once noted that:

> Generally speaking, when people are exposed to numerous and often conflicting messages, as is usually the case, they tend to maintain their established habits. But with well-designed media interventions in appropriate social contexts, significant effects can be achieved. It has been a common experience in the North Karelia Project that such effects may be limited in relative terms, but because of the large audience can be large overall and thus able to generate a very favourable cost-effect ratio.

One antidote to mixed and unhelpful messages is a concerted effort among partnering organizations to agree on and then promote (both individually and jointly) a consistent package of prevention information.

Whatever the ultimate value of mass media, interpersonal channels of communication ought to be considered as well. Indeed, as described in the previous section, the formal dissemination work of community health workers and the more informal approach of lay opinion leaders may be the most effective messaging system of all.

Accessibility Enhancement Methods (Such as Mobile Units)

As described in the previous section, "getting the word out" is one issue in prevention efforts; a complementary challenge is getting the program to the people. Although not part of all the case studies, complementing a CPE-like program with mobile units seems to be a well-accepted approach. Resources such as the Big Bus of Action Cancer in Northern Ireland and the mobile mammography service of British Columbia offer a strategic alternative delivery model for health promotion and screening in rural or other areas where permanent facilities and critical equipment are not available. Responding to accessibility issues could be a key to reducing the disparity in rates of cancer (and other chronic diseases) that is observed in rural and otherwise isolated populations.

The Big Bus shows how far the concept of a mobile unit can be taken. The vehicle incorporates comprehensive program delivery that spans the spectrum of cancer prevention. Its public image reflects a strong brand, one that is sustained through sponsored advertising. The mobile mammography unit in British Columbia has a narrower focus in terms of service delivery, and perhaps has a lower public profile. The prevention educators in both jurisdictions express similar appreciation for the potential to integrate their other work with the scheduled visit of the mobile units to one of their communities. Programs that currently have a mobile unit focusing on screening may want to consider the usefulness of expanding the types of prevention services that are made available in isolated areas.

Having briefly examined the nine identified success factors, two items remain that require more substantial treatment. The next two chapters will cover:

- An important element that typically shapes the planning and launch of a CPE-like program, namely, theory or a conceptual framework
- Evaluation, a component that is customary at the end of a program cycle, although it needs to be incorporated from the start

Sources and Further Reading

Pilot Approach Followed by Program Expansion

van Teijlingen ER, Rennie AM, Hundley V, et al. The importance of conducting and reporting pilot studies: the example of the Scottish Births Survey. J Adv Nurs. 2001;34(3):289–95. http://dx.doi.org/10.1046/j.1365-2648.2001.01757.x. Medline:11328433

van Teijlingen E, Hundley V. The importance of pilot studies. Nurs Stand. 2002;16(40):33–6. Medline:12216297

Comprehensive Targets and Platforms

Matson Koffman D, Granade SA, Anwuri VV. Strategies for establishing policy, environmental, and systems-level interventions for managing high
blood pressure and high cholesterol in health care settings: a qualitative
case study. Prev Chronic Dis. 2008;5(3):A83. Medline:18558033

Plescia M, Young S, Ritzman RL. Statewide community-based health
promotion: a North Carolina model to build local capacity for
chronic disease prevention. Prev Chronic Dis. 2005;2(Spec no):A10.
Medline:16263043

Pronk NP, Peek CJ, Goldstein MG. Addressing multiple behavioral risk factors in primary care. A synthesis of current knowledge and stakeholder
dialogue sessions. Am J Prev Med. 2004;27(2 Suppl):4–17. http://dx.doi.
org/10.1016/j.amepre.2004.04.024. Medline:15275669

Beyond Primary Prevention

Krueger H, McLean D, Williams D. *The Prevention of Second Primary Cancers: A
Resource for Clinicians and Health Managers*. Basel: Karger; 2008.

Veronesi U, Bonanni B. Chemoprevention: from research to clinical oncol-
ogy. Eur J Cancer. 2005;41(13):1833–41. http://dx.doi.org/10.1016/j.
ejca.2005.06.007. Medline:16061373

University Research Partnerships

Best A, Stokols D, Green LW, et al. An integrative framework for community
partnering to translate theory into effective health promotion strategy. Am
J Health Promot. 2003;18(2):168–76. http://dx.doi.org/10.4278/0890-1171-
18.2.168. Medline:14621414

Burdine JN, McLeroy K, Blakely C, et al. Community-based participatory research and community health development. J Prim Prev. 2010;31(1-2):1–7.
http://dx.doi.org/10.1007/s10935-010-0205-9. Medline:20143162

Israel BA, Schulz AJ, Parker EA, et al. Review of community-based research:
assessing partnership approaches to improve public health. Annu Rev Public Health. 1998;19(1):173–202. http://dx.doi.org/10.1146/annurev.publ-
health.19.1.173. Medline:9611617

Letcher AS, Perlow KM. Community-based participatory research shows
how a community initiative creates networks to improve well-being.
Am J Prev Med. 2009;37(6 Suppl 1):S292–9. http://dx.doi.org/10.1016/j.
amepre.2009.08.008. Medline:19896032

Ross LF, Loup A, Nelson RM, et al. The challenges of collaboration for academic and community partners in a research partnership: points to consider. J Empir Res Hum Res Ethics. 2010;5(1):19–32. http://dx.doi.org/10.1525/jer.2010.5.1.19. Medline:20235861

Thompson B, Ondelacy S, Godina R, et al. A small grants program to involve communities in research. J Community Health. 2010;35(3):294–301. http://dx.doi.org/10.1007/s10900-010-9235-8. Medline:20146091

Thompson LS, Story M, Butler G. Use of a university-community collaboration model to frame issues and set an agenda for strengthening a community. Health Promot Pract. 2003;4(4):385–92. http://dx.doi.org/10.1177/1524839903255467. Medline:14611023

Torrence WA, Yeary KH, Stewart C, et al. Evaluating coalition capacity to strengthen community-academic partnerships addressing cancer disparities. J Cancer Educ. 2011;26(4):658–63. http://dx.doi.org/10.1007/s13187-011-0240-0. Medline:21633920

Valente TW, Fujimoto K, Palmer P, et al. A network assessment of community-based participatory research: linking communities and universities to reduce cancer disparities. Am J Public Health. 2010;100(7):1319–25. http://dx.doi.org/10.2105/AJPH.2009.171116. Medline:20466964

Lay Health Advisers

Anderson EE. The role of community-based organizations in the recruitment of human subjects: ethical considerations. Am J Bioeth. 2010;10(3):20–1. http://dx.doi.org/10.1080/15265161003599667. Medline:20229409

Balcázar HG, de Heer H, Rosenthal L, et al. A promotores de salud intervention to reduce cardiovascular disease risk in a high-risk Hispanic border population, 2005–2008. Prev Chronic Dis. 2010;7(2):A28. Medline:20158973

Carr SM, Lhussier M, Forster N, et al. An evidence synthesis of qualitative and quantitative research on component intervention techniques, effectiveness, cost-effectiveness, equity and acceptability of different versions of health-related lifestyle advisor role in improving health. Health Technol Assess. 2011;15(9):iii–iv, 1–284. Medline:21329611

Fleury J, Keller C, Perez A, et al. The role of lay health advisors in cardiovascular risk reduction: a review. Am J Community Psychol. 2009;44(1-2):28–42. http://dx.doi.org/10.1007/s10464-009-9253-9. Medline:19533327

Kash BA, May ML, Tai-Seale M. Community health worker training and certification programs in the United States: findings from a national survey. Health Policy. 2007;80(1):32–42. http://dx.doi.org/10.1016/j.healthpol.2006.02.010. Medline:16569457

Nemcek MA, Sabatier R. State of evaluation: community health workers. Public Health Nurs. 2003;20(4):260–70. http://dx.doi.org/10.1046/j.1525-1446.2003.20403.x. Medline:12823786

O'Brien MJ, Squires AP, Bixby RA, et al. Role development of community health workers: an examination of selection and training processes in the intervention literature. Am J Prev Med. 2009;37(6 Suppl 1):S262–9. Medline:19896028

Plescia M, Newton-Ward M. Increasing the public's awareness: the importance of patient-practitioner communication. N C Med J. 2007;68(5):346–8. Medline:18183757

Story L, Hinton A, Wyatt SB. The role of community health advisors in community-based participatory research. Nurs Ethics. 2010;17(1):117–26. http://dx.doi.org/10.1177/0969733009350261. Medline:20089631

Swider SM. Outcome effectiveness of community health workers: an integrative literature review. Public Health Nurs. 2002;19(1):11–20. http://dx.doi.org/10.1046/j.1525-1446.2002.19003.x. Medline:11841678

Valente TW, Pumpuang P. Identifying opinion leaders to promote behavior change. Health Educ Behav. 2007;34(6):881–96. http://dx.doi.org/10.1177/1090198106297855. Medline:17602096

Media and Marketing Efforts

Abroms LC, Maibach EW. The effectiveness of mass communication to change public behavior. Annu Rev Public Health. 2008;29(1):219–34. http://dx.doi.org/10.1146/annurev.publhealth.29.020907.090824. Medline:18173391

Graham AL, Milner P, Saul JE, et al. Online advertising as a public health and recruitment tool: comparison of different media campaigns to increase demand for smoking cessation interventions. J Med Internet Res. 2008;10(5):e50. http://dx.doi.org/10.2196/jmir.1001. Medline:19073542

Hawn C. Take two aspirin and tweet me in the morning: how Twitter, Facebook, and other social media are reshaping health care. Health Aff (Millwood). 2009;28(2):361–8. http://dx.doi.org/10.1377/hlthaff.28.2.361. Medline:19275991

Maibach EW, Abroms LC, Marosits M. Communication and marketing as tools to cultivate the public's health: a proposed "people and places" framework. BMC Public Health. 2007;7(1):88. http://dx.doi.org/10.1186/1471-2458-7-88. Medline:17519027

Niederdeppe J, Bu QL, Borah P, et al. Message design strategies to raise public awareness of social determinants of health and population health disparities. Milbank Q. 2008;86(3):481–513. http://dx.doi.org/10.1111/ j.1468-0009.2008.00530.x. Medline:18798887

Puska P, Vartiainen E, Laatikainen T, et al. *The North Karelia Project: From North Karelia to National Action*. Helsinki: Helsinki University Printing House; 2009.

Renaud L, Bouchard C, Caron-Bouchard M, et al. A model of mechanisms underlying the influence of media on health behaviour norms. Can J Public Health. 2006;97(2):149–52. Medline:16620006

Thackeray R, Neiger BL, Hanson CL, et al. Enhancing promotional strategies within social marketing programs: use of Web 2.0 social media. Health Promot Pract. 2008;9(4):338–43. http://dx.doi.org/10.1177/1524839908325335. Medline:18936268

Accessibility Enhancement Methods (Such as Mobile Units)

Hartley D. Rural health disparities, population health, and rural culture. Am J Public Health. 2004;94(10):1675–8. http://dx.doi.org/10.2105/ AJPH.94.10.1675. Medline:15451729

Moulavi D, Bushy A, Peterson J, et al. Thinking about a mobile health unit to deliver services? Things to consider before buying. Aust J Rural Health. 2000;8(1):6–16. http://dx.doi.org/10.1046/j.1440-1584.2000.81222.x. Medline:11040574

11 Establishing a Foundation: Conceptual Frameworks

Program theory is a conceptual plan, with some details about what the program is and how it is expected to work ... Whether one is developing a new health program or designing an evaluation for an existing health program, understanding and articulating the program theory is essential.
 – Issel LM. *Health Program Planning and Evaluation* (2008)

This chapter deals with the role of conceptual frameworks or theories in shaping prevention efforts. This theme should be prominent when any health care program is developed; most leaders would agree that understanding and implementing theory is a prerequisite for effective program planning. The following chapter travels to the other end of the planning cycle, the theme of evaluation. Of course, the successful application of theory and evaluation is not restricted to any one point but will instead pervade the entire process; in other words, "feedback loops" are anticipated in both areas. Finally, theory and evaluation can be thought of as two more "important elements" in successful programs involving community-based educators; thus, this chapter and the next will cover in depth two themes that could be added to the inventory found in chapter 10.

The importance of these two topics is reinforced by the fact that they consistently appear in the prevention educator models examined. In particular, a key reason for the focus in the present chapter is that theory was an explicit part of the launch of a community-based prevention educator (CPE) program in British Columbia. Furthermore, theory is of continuing importance according to the key informants from this program; in the survey completed by the CPEs, a large number of theories

Table 11.1 Conceptual Frameworks: Frequency of Mention in CPE Surveys

Health promotion	16
Community engagement	16
Health education	15
Social determinants	15
Population health	13
Community development	11
Community-based research	11
Cultural competency	11

Other: Social inclusion; Ethnic inclusion; First Nations; Health inequities; Community mobilization; Capacity building; Harm reduction; Self-management and efficacy; Healthy communities; Healthy public policy; Urban planning; Human development; Asset-based development.

or conceptual frameworks were identified as influences on their work (see Table 11.1).

In this chapter, after brief introductory comments on theory, two conceptual areas of special interest in CPE-like programs will be explored: *diffusion of innovations* and *health promotion/education*.

Preamble on Theory in Community-Based Prevention

Definition and Examples

A theory in health care is a set of beliefs that guides both thinking and practice. More formally, a theory is composed of abstract statements that describe, explain, and potentially predict the relationships among concepts and events in health care. There are hundreds of such statements in the literature, which have had varying levels of influence across the history of health care. They range from very broad philosophical ideas, such as the perspective in science known as positivism, to more focused concepts, such as "community coalition action theory."

Sometimes theories have been developed in other disciplines and then applied to health care. Complexity theory is a good example; it was first formulated in physics and mathematics, but has since been applied to a wide variety of fields, including health care management. Another example is the theory of communicative action, developed by German philosopher and sociologist Jürgen Habermas and described in two seminal volumes published 30 years ago. This theory had a direct influence on the planning of the pilot CPE program in British Columbia, the Waddell Project. According to the academics involved in the project, the theory developed by Habermas was instrumental in positioning the program as being both *for* and *by* the community. Central to this application were three key "interests" in life as described by Habermas; alternatively, these may be thought of as three different types of knowledge, as follows:

1 Work knowledge: the way one creates and controls the environment
2 Practical knowledge: human social interaction, or social knowledge
3 Emancipatory knowledge: self-knowledge or self-reflection

Academics and planners involved with the Waddell Project believed that traditional cancer prevention programs were particularly weak in promoting the third interest, that is, the type of knowledge that leads to authentic and autonomous personal choices. For this reason, Baillie and other academics attached to the project focused on working with communities to identify the social and other barriers to making healthy choices, and how they could be removed to allow individuals to make those choices more easily on their own. In short, the unhealthy people in a region were considered to be trapped to some extent by socioeconomic factors; given this, the leaders maintained that "the driving force behind the Waddell Project comes from the belief that emancipatory change is central to community health."

The Value of Theory

Adopting or adapting an existing theory or creating a new one is an opportunity to organize thinking about a health care program in a systematic way. In the best situations, it helps to generate an explicit checklist of priorities and related action steps. Because the ideas involved are abstract, a theory helps to explain a plan or strategy in a more general way, so that other leaders can more easily adapt it to their own setting. This aspect of theory is especially important for a research agenda. As was once noted by Verran in a nursing context, "theory-driven investigations are necessary for generalization of findings and development of health care policy." Sometimes practitioners and clients alike are alienated from theory because of confusion about the specialized terminology – the jargon – that is often used; however, in the best scenarios, careful use of language and even coining new terms can help to clarify ideas that ultimately may convey substantial power when put into practice.

The Danger of Theory

The mere attachment of the word "theory" to a concept, although a standard manoeuvre in the academic world, does not automatically add intellectual or practical value. Sometimes it can create a barrier, such as when unnecessary complexity is injected into a perfectly clear and simple idea. An example is the so-called story theory, which is aimed at reminding clinicians that each client has a unique personal and cultural story that needs to be respected. Elevating this self-evident idea to the level of a theory does not seem very helpful, and may even distract from more important issues that need to be clarified and managed.

In a similar vein, a great deal of intellectual effort and planning goes into understanding and embracing "new" theoretical constructs that are very similar to existing ideas. A case in point may be the theory of communicative action noted earlier, a conceptual framework that was influential in the beginning of British Columbia's CPE program. The thought categories proposed by Habermas may be overly subtle for a health care program. Stripped down to its useful features, this theory does not seem appreciably different from other well-accepted ideas in prevention, such as the ecological perspective at the heart of health promotion, the social determinants of health, the vital importance of community engagement, etc. Care must always be taken to avoid getting caught up in abstract language exercises, rather than, for example, simply spending more time paying attention to community members in designing community-based prevention interventions.

One of the greatest dangers of theory applied to health care (and other disciplines) is the existence of an *unacknowledged* theory informing a plan or process. As suggested above, conceptual frameworks can exercise great influence over the priorities and action steps in a health program. Therefore, the theoretical foundation of planning decisions ought to be identified and made transparent to stakeholders. Closely related to the problem of unacknowledged theories, and certainly more common, are *acknowledged* theories that are stated in a way that makes them seem like self-evident laws rather than hypotheses that are still being tested. By definition, a theory is a chosen way of thinking based on beliefs; in other words, it is influenced by ideology. To protect against dogmatism, prevention theories need to be continuously tested by observation and research that supply factual data; as dictated by experimental and real world evaluation, a prevailing theory ought to be modifiable, and even supplantable by a theory that has more explanatory power and potential to create lasting health benefits. In short, theories in the arena of community-based prevention programs should be open to critique, such as the one offered by Forbes and Wainwright on the influential explanations put forward for health inequalities.

This chapter will now turn to two theoretical frameworks that have been especially fruitful in the development of community-based prevention efforts, namely, diffusion of innovations and health promotion. They are both examples of ideas with substantial and well-documented influence, and therefore represent frameworks that ought to be located at the opposite end of the spectrum from frivolous or implicit theories.

Diffusion of Innovations

The origin of the conceptual framework known as the diffusion of innovations (DOI) may be traced to the work of nineteenth-century social scientists such as Gabriel Tarde, Friedrich Ratzel, and Leo Frobenius. It gained momentum as a theory with explanatory power through a 1957 study that tracked the spreading popularity of hybrid corn seed in Iowa and a subsequent book by Everett Rogers entitled *Diffusion of Innovations* (published in 1963). Since then, its principles have been widely adopted and investigated, with well over 5,000 published studies. In a sense, the DOI theory itself has undergone a diffusion process!

In the public health realm, DOI has been embedded in a larger framework known as network analysis. The latter has been used to study: disease transmission, especially related to the human immunodeficiency virus and other sexually transmitted infections; the role of social support and social capital; the influence of personal and social networks on health behaviour; and the structure of prevention health systems. When the networking focus involves information transmission, and especially public health innovations, DOI is most often the specific type of analysis applied.

Rogers defined DOI as *the process by which an innovation is communicated through certain channels over time among the members of a particular social system.* This definition encompasses four dimensions, as described below:

1 An **innovation** is an *idea, practice, or object that is perceived as new by an individual, planning group, etc.* In the case of chronic disease prevention programs, the term could be applied to desirable health behaviours. Although the core idea in itself may not be novel, presenting it alongside new evidence, for example, of the health effects of smoking cessation, could qualify it as an innovation. Because DOI requires that the message be passed between individuals, ensuring that the innovation is relevant and captures the attention of an audience is thought to be a prerequisite for adoption and diffusion.

2 **Communication channels** are the *means by which messages get from one individual to another.* The channels can be broadly categorized into mass media or interpersonal. The use of mass media can be effective at getting the message out. However, interpersonal communication by individuals who influence the opinions and decisions of others is generally considered the most effective way to facilitate adoption of innovations. Intriguingly, the channels of media and word of mouth have been integrated in a dramatic way in the contemporary world through so-called social media; this "hybrid" type of channel has only begun to be exploited by the health care arena, but it is a vehicle in which the CPEs and other leaders in prevention are expressing increasing interest.

3 A **social system** is defined as a *set of interrelated units that are engaged in joint problem solving to accomplish a common goal.* The key, then, is to "recruit" as many such social units – large or small – as possible to work towards the same goal. Some individuals will be naturally aligned with the goals of CPE-like leaders, namely, similar professionals from other agencies and members of the public who have been affected by cancer or other chronic disease. However, the engagement of the social system can be much broader. Potential prevention partners include school administrators and municipal government officials. "Lay" leaders from any sphere ought not to be neglected; while they may not have access to the resources and status reserved for professionals, a formal or informal network of lay leaders can exert an influence through sheer numbers. Figure 11.1 summarizes the channels and social systems that may bear on a DOI process.

4 Over **time**, the innovation diffuses through the social systems by various communication channels, and eventually leads to social change that has a population-wide effect. The rate of adoption is defined as the *relative speed with which an innovation is adopted by members of a social system.*

In the context of community-based prevention, the fundamental aim of DOI is to get out a prevention message as widely as possible and get it accepted as soon as possible. Descriptions of the North Karelia Project explicitly cite DOI as a cornerstone strategy, specifically with respect to the mobilization of lay opinion leaders. As described by Puska and colleagues, these included community members who were "more exposed to mass media, and to social contacts, have higher social status and more influence as a change agent, and show more innovativeness. Opinion leaders are often in a key position to influence wider adoption of an innovation by being themselves satisfied with it and by communicating this opinion through interpersonal networks."

The local Heart Association set up interviews with candidates in various areas of North Karelia. Two opinion leaders were ultimately selected and invited to attend a two-day training seminar. The curriculum included how to respond to the smoking and dietary habits of their neighbours by advising them about behavioural changes and even making referrals to local health professionals.

It is likely that DOI is a formal or informal perspective shared by all lay health adviser programs in the world, including those identified in the Kentucky and North Carolina case studies. But DOI theory extends well beyond the mobilization of lay leaders. For example, work with health care professionals is also vital to community-based prevention efforts. Again, the North Karelia Project modelled this by liaising with physicians, public health nurses, and the leaders of non-profit health organizations.

Ultimately, the forces at work in a DOI process can move a successful or promising initiative beyond the boundaries of the original target area to a broader region and sometimes an entire nation. A good example of this phenomenon is the well-documented diffusion of tobacco control policy throughout North America. Driven by public interest work and advocacy through multiple organizations, tobacco control policy has "leapfrogged." This means that leaders borrow policy from neighbouring jurisdictions and apply it in their area, but often with enhanced features; the original jurisdiction is likely to repeat the process.

Figure 11.1. Potential Pathways in Diffusion of Innovations.

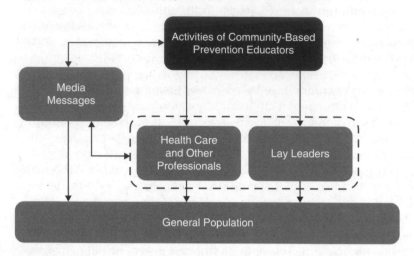

The result has been ever-improving tobacco regulations across all borders, aided by the similarity of culture between Canada and the United States and healthy "competition" among provinces and states within each country.

As suggested above, the principles of DOI may be at work in a program even if they are not explicitly recognized. However, it has become clear that formally acknowledging the DOI theory and strategically incorporating it in all planning stages of a program can enhance the spread and adoption of prevention efforts.

Health Promotion (and Health Education)

Health promotion arguably represents the most prominent conceptual framework influencing CPE-like programs; it may be most accurately seen as an approach comprised of one or more core ideas that are modified by a variety of theories. Along with community engagement, health promotion actually "topped the chart" in terms of the frameworks favoured by CPEs in British Columbia. In fact, there is a strong semantic overlap between health promotion and community engagement, action, or development, as well as concepts such as the socioecologic model, social determinants of health, and healthy communities.

The constellation of ideas represented by this list of near synonyms appears to dominate the thinking within CPE-like programs.

The topic of health education is also often closely connected to health promotion/community action. In fact, both spheres are included as twin pillars in the CPE role description in British Columbia. However, the very fact that they are distinguished in that role description suggests that health promotion and health education should be distinguished.

The balance of this chapter will provide a historical context for public health practice before distinguishing the two spheres of health promotion and education. Finally, some further details about the conceptual framework of health promotion will be provided.

History of Embracing the Social Context Health

The social context of health is not a new idea; it may be traced to at least the 1800s, and the work of researchers and leaders such as German physician Rudolf Virchow (1821–1902). A large part of the motivation for his efforts was concern for the effect of social processes on the health of workers during the Industrial Revolution. The field of study that emerged from this concern became known as social medicine; although some of the thinking was applied to the practice of medicine per se, the ultimate aim was to pursue social changes that could foster a healthier society. Another towering figure, born in Germany less than a year before Virchow, was Friedrich Engels; recognizing the social influence on health and disease was one of the issues that shaped his overall thinking, which famously led to the development of communist theory.

Despite these earlier roots, in the first half of the twentieth century the public health agenda was still dominated by individual behaviour change; dealing with a broader context for health was limited to environmental reforms concerning sanitation and water quality issues. This is in part understandable since, at the population level, communicable diseases of mostly acute onset were the leading causes of morbidity and mortality. Health-seeking behaviour was primarily focused on personal hygiene and increasing uptake of immunization programs; health education efforts were aimed at reinforcing these two priorities.

In the latter half of the twentieth century, chronic diseases displaced infectious conditions as the greatest population health burden. Policymakers were concerned that public health education and personal attempts to change behaviour would not be sufficient to address emerging health issues. The prominent targets were lifestyle factors such as smoking, poor nutrition, and physical inactivity, each representing a complex phenomenon with multiple societal forces at work. Health promotion was born out of the recognition that fostering community empowerment and facilitating collective social action were necessary to change broader societal forces and ultimately create the desired public health impact.

The year 1974 represented a turning point in the history of health promotion. With the publication of Canada's landmark policy statement, *A New Perspective on the Health of Canadians*, and the Health Information and Health Promotion Act passed by the U.S. Congress, health promotion became a significant component of national health policy in North America. Consistent with an appreciation of broader targets was the focus on new platforms of change agency. The scope of health policy and programs began to expand beyond the realm of health institutions to include other sectors of society, from schools and workplaces, to social and family services, to taxation and regulation, to recreation and transportation.

Canada has continued to be at the forefront of the modern focus on a social context for health and disease, and emerging theory and discipline of health promotion. The first international conference on health promotion was hosted in Ottawa in 1986. It produced the very influential document known as the Ottawa Charter, which spelled out the core idea of health promotion, namely that health is "created and lived by people within the settings of their everyday life; where they learn, work, play and love." Two theoretical themes are woven together in this core idea:

- People are responsible for creating health individually and communally; in other words, they have strengths and are meant to be in control of determining their needs and finding solutions to problems
- People need to be supported in their health-creating endeavours, specifically by public policies that lower socioeconomic barriers in order to make the healthy choice the easy choice

The first theme seems very close to the principle of emancipatory knowledge as articulated by Habermas. As noted earlier in the context of the start of the British Columbia CPE program, "the driving force behind the Waddell Project comes from the belief that emancipatory change is central to community health."

The socioeconomic barriers noted in the second theme have become known by the phrase "social determinants" of health. They have been variously identified. In 1998, Health Canada developed the following comprehensive list of determinants of health: income, social support, education and literacy, employment and working conditions, social environments, physical environments, personal health practices and coping skills, healthy child development, biology and genetic endowment, health services, gender, and culture. Since then, the inventory has been narrowed to the *social* determinants of health. This scoping work culminated in the 2008 report by the World Health Organization's Commission on Social Determinants of Health, which delineated this smaller, somewhat overlapping inventory of social categories, or conditions of daily living:

- Equitable start in life (including supports in early childhood and universal education)
- Fair employment and decent work
- Healthy urban and rural places
- Social protection across the life course
- Universal health care

This list is interesting as much for what it includes as for what it does not include. There appears to have been a desire to avoid headlining some of the classic categories of social concern, such as poverty or income and decent and/or affordable housing, and instead use novel ways to express the same ideas. However the list of social determinants may be refined in the future, these sorts of categories represent the key targets of health promotion work.

Promotion versus Education

Health promotion and health education are obviously related, in that they are both concerned with health, and share certain underlying theoretical foundations. But the two spheres are different. Whitehead, writing from a nursing perspective, has been particularly helpful in distinguishing health promotion and education. Health education may be defined as follows:

> An activity that seeks to inform the individual on the nature and causes of health/illness and that individual's personal level of risk associated with

their lifestyle-related behaviour. Health education seeks to motivate the individual to accept a process of behavioural change through directly influencing their value, belief and attitude systems, where it is deemed that the individual is particularly at risk or has already been affected by illness/disease or disability.

Thus, it seems that health education generally targets an at-risk individual, but the educational setting and audience conceivably could be a formal or informal group. Health promotion by definition exists at the other end of the audience spectrum, aiming at population-level changes in structures, resources, and, ultimately, health. In short, health promotion has a broader focus on community empowerment, rather than simply targeting individuals who need to change their risky behaviours. It may be defined as follows:

> Health promotion is the process by which the ecologically-driven socio-political-economic determinants of health are addressed as they impact on individuals and the communities within which they interact ... Health promotion seeks to radically transform and empower communities through involving them in activities that influence their public health – particularly via agenda setting, political lobbying and advocacy, critical consciousness-raising and social education programs.

The confusion between the two spheres of education and promotion may be traceable to the core idea of health promotion as described earlier, and the embedded themes of personal empowerment and social change. The fact is that an educational component can be posited across such an agenda (see Figure 11.2), with individuals and groups as the audience on one side and community organization leaders and broader policy-makers as the audience on the other side.

Furthermore, considering that personal empowerment (one of the avowed goals of health promotion) can certainly be fostered by learning, health education has a direct role to play in advancing the cause of health promotion. In this way, it may be best to consider health education as a subset of health promotion. This conclusion is strengthened by the acknowledgment that health education activities, when pursued intensively and extensively across a jurisdiction, can contribute to the sort of population-level effects that are the ultimate aim of health promotion. It is arguable that this very pattern and outcome was seen in the North Karelia Project, which sponsored hundreds of health education

Figures 11.2. Approaches to Health-Related Practice:
Health Education vs. Health Promotion.

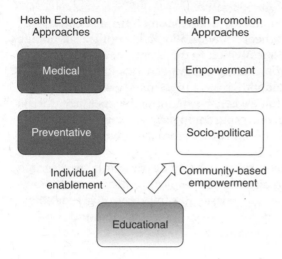

encounters over the years. However, for all of their overlaps, it may still be advisable to distinguish between health promotion and health education. Although the value of health education may need to be re-asserted today, the fact is that teaching individuals is an easier assignment than changing communities and whole societies. There has been a tendency in some quarters for health promotion work to devolve to health education; the broader focus on social determinants must be maintained by preserving the true definition of health promotion.

Promotion versus Programs

The implications of a strategy that is too focused on health-related programs can be very subtle. A program delivery orientation exists in a certain degree of tension with the classic "bottom-up" approach that involves identifying needs and generating tailored responses through community collaboration. The challenge comes when programs are not completely "on target" in terms of local priorities, and thus have a poor track record of community uptake. Such obstacles can be discouraging for the CPE and the community alike. Even when there are positive effects, the time required to adapt and administer a program takes away from opportunities for local innovation. Nonetheless, centrally managed programs can have their place, as long as the advantages are maximized and the downsides are mitigated.

One upside of a program created and resourced from "head office" is that "reinvention of the wheel" may be avoided. Another advantage is that resources are automatically tied to the program, without having to raise funds for a new approach; this saves energy for both prevention educators and stakeholders. As well, high-quality materials can be produced that help to reinforce a consistent, attractive message. Media tie-ins to multiple offerings of a program in different regions can create momentum across a jurisdiction; in other words, it is easier to spread a "brand" that is well-known.

The downside of top-down programs can be mitigated by a certain degree of local adaption, a careful process of introduction that allows for better community buy-in. In general, it is important to ensure there are not too many such offerings to manage, so that leaders and community members do not become fatigued.

Applications of Health Promotion in Model Programs

During the conception of the pilot Waddell Project in British Columbia, its designers identified and responded to a number of challenges that had faced previous community-based programs aimed at health promotion, as follows:

- Rather than using an individual focus, shift to a collaborative vision of how health beliefs and decisions are imprinted on an entire community; leverage this renewed understanding to change the environment, and remove barriers in order to make healthy choices the easy choices
- Recognize that information strategies are not sufficient to change the underlying behaviour, partly because one is competing with a lot of information, including *misinformation*; in addition, knowing better does not automatically mean doing better
- In light of the preceding point, it is important to ensure that the flow of information is bilateral, allowing for mutual enlightenment of student and educator
- Recognize that time is essential for any centrally designed program to be refined and tailored specifically for a target community;

evaluation of the program and solving problems that arise will increase community support and the potential for effectiveness

The health promotion aspect of the initial CPE program in British Columbia was operationalized through a sequence of carefully designed stages, as follows:

1 Approach the municipal council and request permission to launch the Waddell Project
2 Community members introduced to the project through interaction with community organizations, talks given at events, local media exposure, etc. – all aimed at creating a foundation of trust
3 Call on the connections made in the first stages to bring together key individuals and representatives of local groups to discuss their community, the challenges they face, etc.
4 From this pool, form a steering committee of 8–12 people. The committee develops an interview questionnaire for the community, to be answered by individuals and small groups
5 Advertise for and hire a community-based prevention educator to act as the health promotion agent
6 The British Columbia Cancer Agency's Centre for the Southern Interior (CSI) shifts to a supportive role
7 Design, implement, and evaluate community-determined health promotion initiatives, with continued support from CSI

There appears to have been a classic health promotion framework in the pilot work conducted in the interior of British Columbia. It is an open question whether that pattern has been maintained at the same level as the program expanded across the province in more recent years. The fact that a committee had to be struck to explore a focus on social determinants in the province suggests that it may be an area for ongoing renewal.

As noted earlier, one of the explicit roles of British Columbia's CPEs is so-called public education; this is accomplished directly through presentations that align with the knowledge base and skill set of the particular CPE. In reality, CPEs are always in a teaching role, no matter what the occasion may be. Even in committee or coalition meetings, a CPE will seek to bring relevant information to bear on the discussion.

Table 11.2 Components of Prevention Educator Programs

Case Study	Health Education	Health Promotion
Northern Ireland	√	
North Karelia	√	√
North Carolina (CHAP)	√	
Kentucky HEEL	√	√
Kentucky KCP	√	√
Manitoba	√	√
British Columbia CPEs	√	√

As indicated in Table 11.2, the other community-based prevention educator programs discussed all demonstrate a health education component, with less consistent presence of other elements of health promotion.

In North Karelia, educational initiatives directed at the individual included the distribution of informational pamphlets and the presentation of nutrition lectures, with the latter sometimes attached to club meetings, cooking demonstrations, etc. North Karelia also had a significant mass media campaign, a type of health communication even though not qualifying as classic health education. As another example, lay health educators are a key component of health education in the Kentucky Cancer Program; they are trained to reach out to individuals (notably, through home visits) to educate on screening and lifestyle choices.

Despite the fact that the term "health promotion" appears in the job title in Northern Ireland, the program does not meet the classic definition of health promotion. The health promotion officers in that jurisdiction provide services mostly on an individual basis; community collaborations or policy-related initiatives focusing on broader determinants of health are absent from the assignment. In North Carolina, the community health ambassadors work on a one-to-one basis and at present do not engage in community action. The remaining case studies clearly point to health promotion activities; this is usually apparent in the stated objectives of the program, including terms such as: community collaboration, mobilization, or empowerment; social action; and environmental change. The North Karelia Project and its expanded version throughout Finland demonstrated the widest range of health promotion activities, from community-level by-laws to lobbying food processing companies to national-level policy changes.

Principles of Health Promotion Practice

A program using the strategy of community-based prevention educators ought to consider the degree of commitment to classic health promotion called for by its mandate or vision statement, and to honestly evaluate how much the theoretical underpinnings of health promotion are informing its activities. If, on analysis, health education is the dominant motif in practice, then that reality ought to be acknowledged; in such instances, the job title "health promotion officer" should not be used; it is arguable that "community-based prevention educator" would also not be a very accurate label under such circumstances.

If, however, health promotion theory and activities are explicitly on the agenda, then a number of principles should be regularly reviewed. These include the following points:

- Health promotion has a long history, and it involves complex perspectives and choice of influential conceptual frameworks; inservice training and refreshers on health promotion theory and practice ought to be built in to any CPE program. To quote University of Toronto Public Health Professor Cameron Norman, "health promotion's focus on the multilayered, complex interactions that create or limit health and wellbeing require knowledge and action that match this complexity."
- Health promotion is by definition comprehensive, involving multiple targets and platforms. This is illustrated very well in Figure 11.3. A comprehensive plan that matches the breadth of these concerns should be in place.
- As well as not being consumed by a health education model, it is important that CPEs not be solely occupied with delivery of centrally designed programs. Programs can be very useful, especially when there is freedom and opportunity to adapt them, but if there is little space left over to create community-designed solutions the principles and potential of true health promotion will be compromised.
- Time and energy must be protected to allow the strategic activities of true health promotion to flourish, such as identifying and

Figure 11.3. Typology of Health Promotion: Activities.

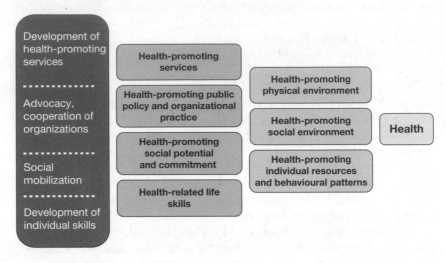

gathering organizational key stakeholders, articulating barriers and challenges, assessing needs and assets, working with partners to build evidence-based services, funding and budgeting, evaluation, advocacy (as appropriate), and professional development.

The preceding discussion of the importance of conceptual frameworks and theory in the work of community-based prevention educators may seem daunting and perhaps even a distraction. In the press of urgent needs and limited hours, there will always be a temptation to short-change the theory component of prevention work. Issel, writing in the 2008 textbook, *Health Program Planning and Evaluation*, offers this warning against such sentiments:

> The theory development phase of program planning requires thinking rather than doing, so it often receives less attention than is needed to fully develop an effective health program. However, using a systematic approach to develop a program theory and to engage stakeholders in the development of the theory has big and long-term payoffs that outweigh any delay or costs associated with developing the theory.

The next chapter will address another area that is sometimes neglected in CPE-like programs, namely, evaluation.

Sources and Further Reading

Theory in Prevention Programs

Alderson P. Theories in health care and research: the importance of theories in health care. BMJ. 1998;317(7164):1007–10. http://dx.doi.org/10.1136/bmj.317.7164.1007. Medline:9765175

Baillie L, Bassett-Smith J, Broughton S. Using communicative action in the primary prevention of cancer. Health Educ Behav. 2000;27(4):442–53. http://dx.doi.org/10.1177/109019810002700407. Medline:10929752

Baillie L, Broughton S, Bassett-Smith J, et al. Community health, community involvement, and community empowerment: too much to expect? J Community Psychol. 2004;32(2):217–28. http://dx.doi.org/10.1002/jcop.10084.

Crosby R, Noar SM. Theory development in health promotion: are we there yet? J Behav Med. 2010;33(4):259–63. http://dx.doi.org/10.1007/s10865-010-9260-1. Medline:20379800

Forbes A, Wainwright SP. On the methodological, theoretical and philosophical context of health inequalities research: a critique. Soc Sci Med. 2001;53(6):801–16. http://dx.doi.org/10.1016/S0277-9536(00)00383-X. Medline:11511055

Green J. The role of theory in evidence-based health promotion practice. Health Educ Res. 2000;15(2):125–9. http://dx.doi.org/10.1093/her/15.2.125. Medline:10751371

Issel LM. *Health Program Planning and Evaluation: A Practical and Systematic Approach for Community Health.* Sudbury, Massachusetts: Jones & Barlett Learning; 2008.

Verran JA. The value of theory-driven (rather than problem-driven) research. Semin Nurse Manag. 1997;5(4):169–72. Medline:9460474

Diffusion of Innovations

Haider M, Kreps GL. Forty years of diffusion of innovations: utility and value in public health. J Health Commun. 2004;9(sup1 Suppl 1):3–11. http://dx.doi.org/10.1080/10810730490271430. Medline:14960400

Hall DM, Escoffery C, Nehl E, et al. Spontaneous diffusion of an effective skin cancer prevention program through Web-based access to program materials. Prev Chronic Dis. 2010;7(6):A125. Medline:20950532

Luke DA, Harris JK. Network analysis in public health: history, methods, and applications. Annu Rev Public Health. 2007;28(1):69–93. http://dx.doi. org/10.1146/annurev.publhealth.28.021406.144132. Medline:17222078

Puska P, Koskela K, McAlister A, et al. Use of lay opinion leaders to promote diffusion of health innovations in a community programme: lessons learned from the North Karelia project. Bull World Health Organ. 1986;64(3):437–46. Medline:3490321

Studlar DT. Diffusion of tobacco control in North America. Ann Am Acad Pol Soc Sci. 1999;566(1):68–79. http://dx.doi.org/10.1177/000271629956600 1006.

Valente TW, Fosados R. Diffusion of innovations and network segmentation: the part played by people in promoting health. Sex Transm Dis. 2006;33(7 Suppl):S23–31. http://dx.doi.org/10.1097/01.olq.0000221018.32533.6d. Medline:16794552

Health Promotion and Health Education

Fertman CI. DD Allensworth, editor. *Health Promotion Programs: From Theory to Practice*. Hoboken, New Jersey: Jossey-Bass; 2010.

Green LW, Kreuter MW. Health promotion as a public health strategy for the 1990s. Annu Rev Public Health. 1990;11(1):319–34. http://dx.doi. org/10.1146/annurev.pu.11.050190.001535. Medline:2191664

Green J, Tones K. *Health Promotion: Planning and Strategies*. 2nd ed. London, UK: SAGE; 2010.

Hay DI. *Economic Arguments for Action on the Social Determinants of Health*. 2006. Available at http://cprn.org/documents/46128_fr.pdf (accessed 28 August 2012).

Irwin A, Scali E. Action on the social determinants of health: a historical perspective. Glob Public Health. 2007;2(3):235–56. http://dx.doi. org/10.1080/17441690601106304. Medline:19283626

Kemm J. Health education: a case for resuscitation. Public Health. 2003;117(2):106–11. http://dx.doi.org/10.1016/S0033-3506(02)00013-6. Medline:12802976

Marmot M, Wilkinson RG, editors. *Social Determinants of Health*. Oxford: Oxford University Press; 2006.

Minkler M, Wallerstein N. Improving health through community organization and community building. In: M Minkler, editor. *Community Organizing and Community Building for Health*. 2nd ed. New Brunswick, New Jersey: Rutgers University Press; 2004.

Norman CD. Health promotion as a systems science and practice. J
    Eval Clin Pract. 2009;15(5):868–72. http://dx.doi.org/10.1111/j.1365-
    2753.2009.01273.x. Medline:19811602

Whitehead D. Health promotion and health education viewed as symbi-
    otic paradigms: bridging the theory and practice gap between them.
    J Clin Nurs. 2003;12(6):796–805. http://dx.doi.org/10.1046/j.1365-
    2702.2003.00804.x. Medline:14632972

Whitehead D. Health promotion and health education: advancing the con-
    cepts. J Adv Nurs. 2004;47(3):311–20. http://dx.doi.org/10.1111/j.1365-
    2648.2004.03095.x. Medline:15238126

World Health Organization. *Closing the Gap in a Generation: Health Equity
    through Action on the Social Determinants of Health*. 2008. Available at http://
    www.who.int/social_determinants/thecommission/finalreport/en/index.
    html (accessed 23 January 2010).

World Health Organization. *Equity, Social Determinants and Public Health
    Programmes*. 2010. Available at http://whqlibdoc.who.int/publica-
    tions/2010/9789241563970_eng.pdf (accessed 23 January 2010) .

12   Tracking Outcomes: Evaluation Matters

The only real challenge in my work is trying to understand how effective and lasting my efforts are. I often wonder have I really made a difference? Has anyone made a change in their life habits or routines? Are there better ways of achieving our objectives than I'm doing now?

— British Columbia prevention educator

Evaluation is being covered in this penultimate chapter because of its great importance to health care in general and its frequent mention in the British Columbia story and in the case studies of other jurisdictions. The comments made by key informants will be reviewed before the topic of evaluation is unpacked in more general terms.

Reports from the Field

Even without the other case studies, information from British Columbia offers a compelling argument for the importance of evaluation as a topic. After the issue of time pressures, evaluation was the most frequent area identified as a program challenge and/or an area of potential improvement.

Among the other case studies, evaluation was also commonly recognized as a very important aspect of a community-based prevention program. Despite this, most programs have minimal evaluation systems in place, and every informant recognized that much more needs to be done. For example, the Brandon Regional Health Authority (RHA) of Manitoba is endeavouring to measure actual behaviour change; although the leaders do gather information on how many people attend a program and how useful it is, they are still trying to enhance this type of "soft" process evaluation with a risk factor survey that could track before-and-after effects. Why do robust evaluation systems focusing on population-level behaviour or disease outcomes take so long to develop? A key informant from this RHA suggested that senior management are sufficiently impacted when they hear anecdotes about individuals being helped, so there may be little motivation to add quantitative outcome data to the qualitative information that is already available. In Interlake, another Manitoba RHA, very little evaluation work has been done as yet, although the informant from the region stated that it remained a "work in progress." The leaders there would ultimately like to be able to incorporate "hard" evaluation data into the feedback they provide to the community, policy-makers, and funders.

The Kentucky Cancer Program (KCP) relies on the behavioural risk factor survey managed by the Centers for Disease Control and Prevention. The results are used to gauge the progress being made across the state from year to year. Cancer incidence and mortality rates are available by county and also in aggregate form by district; this information is used to determine the target population that should be a focus of their programs, allowing the KCP to calibrate efforts in each region. Regular risk factor surveillance guided by national standards and conducted at the local level is certainly valuable, but it still is only a piece of the evaluation picture. The KCP does not appear to have an in-house evaluation protocol that attempts to measure the effect of their overall program or specific strategies. In addition to the effect of secular trends, there are multiple health-promoting organizations in Kentucky that implement various types of prevention interventions. As is often the case with diseases generated by common risk factors, attributing short-term behaviour change or long-term health outcomes to any single program is a very complex task.

Although the Community Health Ambassadors Program (CHAP) in North Carolina is not as comprehensive as the strategies examined in the other case studies, evaluation is just as vital. In fact, it is sometimes easier to link outcomes to an intervention of more limited scope. CHAP's efforts primarily involve lay health education encounters with individuals and small groups. Evaluation is fully integrated by means of surveys administered to people before and after such encounters. Data from the Client Assessment Tool is being analysed by a university research department that is under contract, with the aim of evaluating the impact of the CHAP intervention. Although this tool is not designed to measure population-level effects, it is important to recognize that intensive work with individuals by lay health advisers can eventually add up to a community-wide impact, especially if the effect of the messages is multiplied through the mechanism known as diffusion of innovations (see chapter 11).

North Karelia Project

The notable exception to the pattern of modest evaluation plans may be found in the North Karelia Project, which incorporated a comprehensive evaluation component for both the intervention processes and the intermediate and ultimate health outcomes. This commitment of resources, planning, and personnel (especially university-level researchers) was established from the start. The evaluation program was very comprehensive, as suggested by the following summary provided by Puska and other leaders of the North Karelia Project:

> The aim of the evaluation of the program was to assess the feasibility, effect, costs, process, and other consequences of the program in the community during the 5-year period. The feasibility evaluation should reveal if the intended activities can be established. It should show whether the existing health service resources can be mobilized to serve the program purposes ... The program effect assessment in the North Karelia project was based on large cross-sectional sample surveys in the intervention area and the reference area population at the outset (spring 1972), and at the end of the 5-year period (spring 1977). The program effect was defined as the net reduction in disease and risk factor levels in North Karelia (the reduction in North Karelia minus the reduction in the reference area).

Apart from the general sense of comprehensiveness, the evaluation design suggested here demonstrates a number of features:

1 The prerequisite of understanding something about intervention components *before* they are launched – the evidence base for choosing prevention interventions is of course much larger today than would have existed in the 1970s
2 A commitment to track "hard" outcome data as well as "soft" process information (these terms will be defined more fully later in this chapter) from the start and at every stage

3 A commitment to track financial information, allowing for some level of economic analysis
4 A clear time frame for the pilot investigation, long enough to allow trends to solidify and early signs of disease reduction to be detected
5 Having a clear plan for data collection that is feasible, with structures in place to ensure that it will actually be pursued over the long term
6 The principle of getting good baseline information in the populations of interest, which again speaks to the need to have an evaluation plan in place before the program launches
7 Creating as close to an experimental design as possible, which ultimately permits a fair comparison between intervention and reference or control groups

The last feature is especially important because it is aimed at taking into account the confounding effect of secular trends, that is, the change in risk factor rates or disease incidence that would have happened even if the program had not been put in place. The main challenge of an experimental design that is not based on a fully randomized control approach is locating populations that are reasonably comparable. In the North Karelia Project, a neighbouring province was chosen as the reference area because of its similarities to North Karelia in terms of cardiovascular disease mortality and morbidity, geography, occupational profile, and other socioeconomic characteristics. Cross-sectional surveying of a random sample was chosen instead of longitudinal follow-up of a set cohort; the concern with a longitudinal approach was that the anticipation of the follow-up survey by participants would itself introduce a confounding factor.

Factors such as sample size and age range were carefully considered when conducting each survey; the data collection at the start and end of the study period occurred at the same time of year in both regions. The surveys were mostly self-administered, with any biomarker measurements carried out by specially trained nurses. The same laboratory was used for all serum analyses, and randomly selected samples were sent to a different laboratory for verification of results.

Reflecting on the initial pilot period in North Karelia, Puska and colleagues summed up the importance of program design and evaluation in terms of the eventual application of results to future projects and new jurisdictions: "It is … important that the whole package be designed for possible application on a larger scale in other areas or to the whole country. The results obtained in a community program are ... bound by time, place, and situation. However, through careful and comprehensive evaluation, the meaningfulness of the situation as well as the effects of different intervention components can be discussed and interpreted." As noted more than once in this book, one of the key reasons the North Karelia Project has enjoyed such a remarkable influence in the public health arena around the world is the deep commitment of the program leaders to the discipline of evaluation. There may have been unique conditions in that part of Finland 40 years ago, including the lack of "competing" public health programs to confound any results, but the unique outcomes that were consistently tracked in the project ought to spur on a similar commitment to evaluation in projects today.

Along with the development and application of theory (as discussed in the previous chapter), it seems clear from the "real world" examples that evaluation deserves to be added to the inventory of important program elements or success factors found in chapter 10. The balance of the present chapter provides an overview of the literature on this topic, to guide the evaluation agenda that ought to be considered by any CPE-like program.

Principles Relevant to Evaluation in a CPE-like Program

Cross-cutting Principles

There are a number of "meta principles" that cut across all types of evaluation related to CPE-like strategies. These principles, as laid out below, were found prominently in the case studies and in the literature.

   Principle 1. An evaluation plan needs to be in place from the start, and should be integrated into all stages of the planning process.
   This principle was reinforced in the World Health Organization (WHO) publication *Evaluation in Health Promotion*, as follows:

   Evaluation is inextricably related to and depends on a clear understanding of the conceptual framework underlying the initiative and the processes and elements involved in planning it...the evaluation of health promotion initiatives will only be as good as the preceding planning.

   Principle 2. Resources for data collection and analysis need to be sufficient and sustained.

One of the recommendations for evaluation offered by Israel and colleagues is to "assess outcomes over appropriately long periods of time to determine their persistence." Also, because of the reality of disease latency and slow progression, it is important that the required resources are in place for data collection over the long term so that health outcome effects may be observed.

Principle 3. Community members/stakeholders should be included at all stages of the evaluation process.

Evaluation in health promotion, apart from its other benefits, is a substantial means of empowering individuals and communities. As stated in the WHO publication noted above, community participation in evaluation processes "helps to identify the views of stakeholders, especially the less powerful, increases appreciation of the purpose of the evaluation and understanding and acceptance of the findings, and promotes commitment to act on them." It can also motivate the development of networks and contacts, while providing feedback to the parties involved about the quality of their collaboration. Finally, the involvement of community members in evaluation helps to keep the process honest; the reporting of results should make sense to "end user" clients, and inspire them to make personal changes that will be a model for the rest of the community.

Principle 4. Evaluation reports need to have a clear, practical format suitable for various stakeholders: funders; policy-makers; community groups; prevention team members; media workers; the public; etc.

Dissemination of evaluation findings and recommendations is a fundamental step in the evaluation process. As discussed above, such information is instrumental in empowering individuals and communities; when done effectively from the earliest phases, it can also help to avoid additional resource-intensive evaluation. The importance of disseminating information and presenting the evaluation findings in an appropriate format is highlighted as follows in the WHO publication cited earlier:

> Guidance should be disseminated not only on evaluation but also on how practitioners can make the best use of it. Such a process will affect quality standards in the execution of programmes, so that practitioners may realize the same benefit as the evaluated programmes they wish to replicate. Thus, developing a marketing or dissemination plan should be a required

activity for most, if not all, evaluations of health promotion interventions. It has even been suggested that the effort and resources devoted to disseminating evaluation findings and recommendations should match those spent on creating them.

Principles Related to Prevention Categories

As described in the previous chapter, community-based prevention educators are fundamentally concerned with prevention activities that fall under the umbrella of health promotion. There are three "category principles" that emerge from the literature on the evaluation of health promotion programs; these three concepts, considered in the order they are described below, represent an increasing rigour of program evaluation.

Principle 5. Because the arena of health promotion is multifaceted, it entails many different components requiring evaluation.

Three key facets or application points of health promotion may be identified: the physical environment, the social environment, and people exposed to the program. The full impact in each sphere ought to be evaluated, as well as the process and more immediate impacts related to key health promotion activities. Finally, health outcomes relevant to individual participants in the prevention program need to be considered. The range of evaluation levels and concerns is reflected in Figure 12.1, which is an elaboration of a paradigm introduced in an earlier discussion of health promotion.

Principle 6. Numbers are important in the assessment of prevention programs, but evaluation should also be about the stories. Qualitative evaluation can provide important feedback and inspiration for gatekeepers, field workers, and the community as a whole.

Sometimes the objective numbers will be most important, and sometimes the stories of a program's impact will have the greatest effect. Both types of data are valuable, however, and should be collected and analysed rigorously. Sometimes the two may be merged profitably. Statistics can be made more meaningful by the addition of ordinary human descriptions of a program's impact. Likewise, as noted by Barbour, "qualitative work can be enhanced by using quantitative techniques – albeit often in a modified form – in analysing data, developing sampling strategies, and amalgamating findings from separate qualitative

Figures 12.1. Typology of Health Promotion: Evaluation.

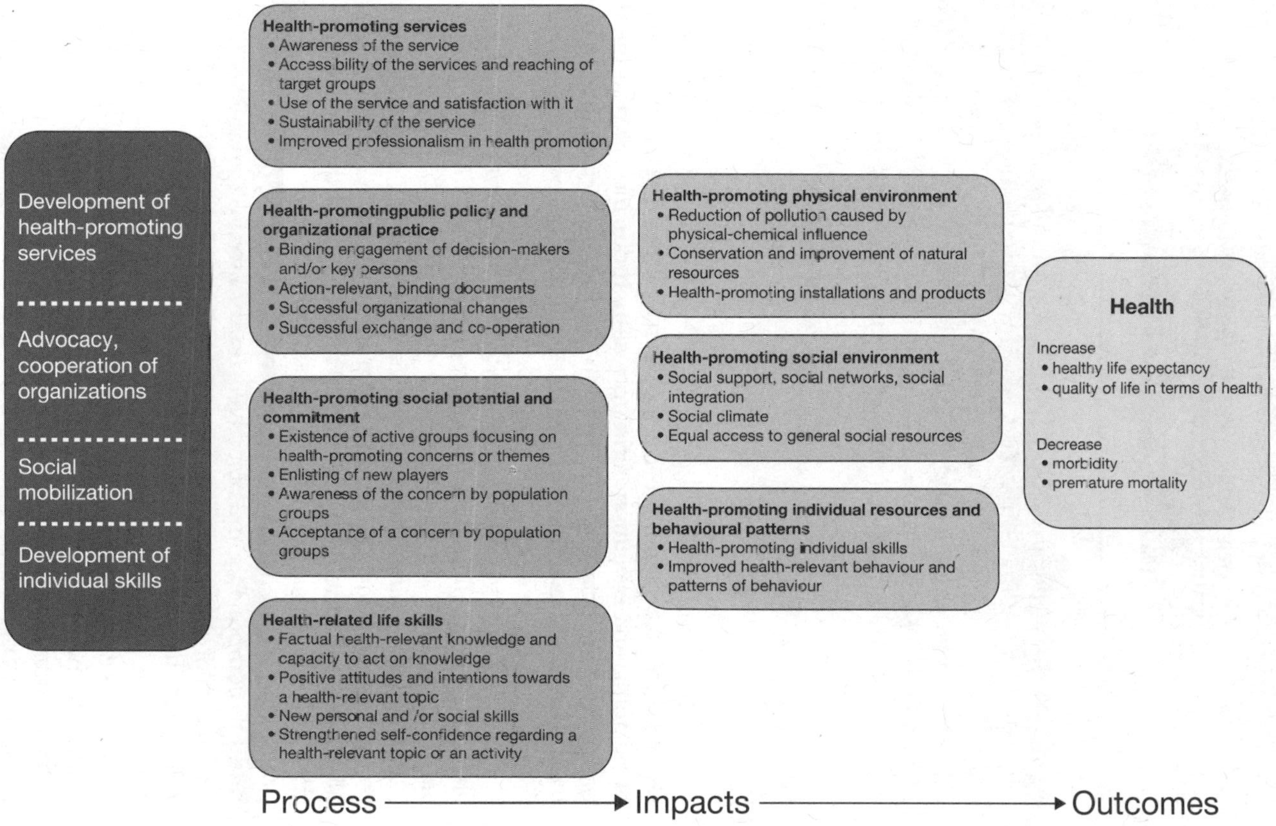

Health-promoting services
- Awareness of the service
- Accessibility of the services and reaching of target groups
- Use of the service and satisfaction with it
- Sustainability of the service
- Improved professionalism in health promotion

Health-promoting public policy and organizational practice
- Binding engagement of decision-makers and/or key persons
- Action-relevant, binding documents
- Successful organizational changes
- Successful exchange and co-operation

Health-promoting social potential and commitment
- Existence of active groups focusing on health-promoting concerns or themes
- Enlisting of new players
- Awareness of the concern by population groups
- Acceptance of a concern by population groups

Health-related life skills
- Factual health-relevant knowledge and capacity to act on knowledge
- Positive attitudes and intentions towards a health-relevant topic
- New personal and /or social skills
- Strengthened self-confidence regarding a health-relevant topic or an activity

Health-promoting physical environment
- Reduction of pollution caused by physical-chemical influence
- Conservation and improvement of natural resources
- Health-promoting installations and products

Health-promoting social environment
- Social support, social networks, social integration
- Social climate
- Equal access to general social resources

Health-promoting individual resources and behavioural patterns
- Health-promoting individual skills
- Improved health-relevant behaviour and patterns of behaviour

Health

Increase
- healthy life expectancy
- quality of life in terms of health

Decrease
- morbidity
- premature mortality

Development of health-promoting services

Advocacy, cooperation of organizations

Social mobilization

Development of individual skills

Process ⟶ Impacts ⟶ Outcomes

Figure 12.2. Program Evaluation Categories.

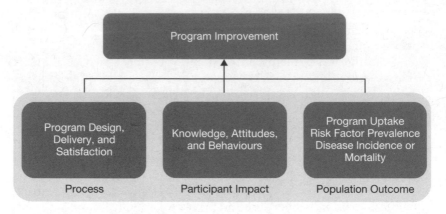

studies." In short, qualitative evaluation still requires rigour in terms of planning and execution; although, as Barbour indicated in another paper, it is important to not develop protocols or checklists that are overzealous and therefore counterproductive.

Principle 7. It is possible to focus solely on monitoring a program's impact on participants and miss evaluating its population-level outcomes. Population outcomes should be on the agenda.

Figure 12.2 outlines three categories or levels of evaluation that may be implemented in a prevention program.

Process evaluation is a natural starting point and the most common type of evaluation found in public health. It focuses on how the program is delivered and how it is received. This type of evaluation has multiple components and objectives. It seeks to:

- Describe the program design and activities
- Elucidate internal dynamics of program operations
- Compare with standards to provide for quality assurance
- Outline the extent of participant exposure
- Identify and describe participants
- Measure provider and participant satisfaction

Participant impact evaluation assesses the program's effectiveness in achieving the desired changes in knowledge, attitudes, beliefs, and behaviours among individuals in the target group. In this category, qualitative results may be as useful as quantitative; however, objective assessments are certainly possible, such as the sort of before-and-after surveys developed by Plescia and others for lay health adviser programs. When proportions are being tracked (e.g., the rate of satisfied clients, or fraction of people who have made behavioural changes), then the denominator is the total number of program participants.

Population outcome evaluation, on the other hand, focuses on the effect of the program on risk factor prevalence, disease incidence, etc. in a region; the denominator in that case becomes the total population. Participant impact evaluation is particularly important when effects on the population are expected to mostly occur over the long term. Thus, the effect of a program on behaviours such as smoking may be measured in the short term, but any effect on lung cancer rates would not manifest itself for many years. This is why tracking risk factor prevalence is so important across the life of a prevention program.

Principle 8. It is possible to remain too "soft" or "superficial" in the population-level impacts that are measured. It is important to evaluate as deeply as possible at any particular phase of a program.

It is certainly useful to measure the proportion of a population that takes advantage of a prevention program, that is, the uptake rate. It is especially relevant when there is almost a one-to-one association between program exposure and ultimate effectiveness, as is seen with certain immunizations. However, it is usually necessary to go beyond the most proximate measurement of uptake to metrics that are further along the population outcome spectrum. Changes in disease incidence and mortality are the "holy grail" of primary and secondary prevention, respectively, but chronic conditions by definition can take a long time to develop; in other words, this type of evaluation requires a long view and, as suggested under Principle 2 above, sustained resources. Prior to the ultimate results unfolding, it is good to understand how a program is affecting risk factor exposure in a population or, in the case of screening, the degree to which disease precursors are being detected and treated. The various population outcome categories are summarized in Table 12.1.

Table 12.1 Population Outcome of a Prevention Program

Outcome Category	Measure
A. Proximate	Uptake Rate = Exposure to a Program
B. Intermediate	1. Risk Factor Prevalence
	2. Disease Precursor Detection Rate
C. Ultimate	1. Disease Incidence
	2. Disease Mortality

A Final Principle

The most common characteristic observed in the discussion with informants from around the world concerning the topic of evaluation was a
sense of inertia. There is a gap between the ideals laid out in the literature for program evaluation and actual practice. This reality points to
the multiple barriers faced by evaluators of prevention programs.

In an assessment of the quality of program evaluations conducted
in South Australian community health services, the main promoters
and the concomitant barriers to evaluation were identified; these are
listed in Table 12.2, according to the frequency of mention by survey
respondents.

This analysis leads naturally to the final principle to be articulated in
this chapter.

*Principle 9. There must be a constantly renewed commitment among pre-
vention program leaders to encourage the promoters of and overcome the barriers to prevention program evaluation.*

Ultimately, there are several reasons to be committed to program
evaluation in as robust a way as possible. Some of the potential advantages are as follows:

- Encouraging funders, policy-makers, and other gatekeepers to continue supporting a program, especially in the face of constrained
  health care resources
- Motivation for field workers, community organizers, etc. to keep up
  the effort
- Facilitating the recruitment of other partners

Table 12.2 Promoters and Barriers to Evaluation (In order of response frequency)

Promoters	Barriers
Skills and training	Not enough time/resources for evaluation
Culture of evaluation	Lack of evaluation culture
Evaluation process or structure	Not enough expertise within organization to do evaluation
Evaluation used to make a difference	Evaluation results aren't used
Access to expertise and support	External evaluation too expensive
Appropriate data systems and evaluation tools	Evaluation not seen as relevant/ appropriate to work
Consistent framework	Evaluation is perceived as a threat to individual or program
Feedback and follow up	Don't know how to interpret evaluation findings

Source: Jolley et al., *Australian Health Review*, 2007.

- Development of reports that will provide compelling content for complementary media campaigns that may contribute to the diffusion of innovations
- Highlighting strengths and weaknesses of a program, in order to understand why the goals were or were not achieved and to assist in replicating the program elsewhere
- Fostering feedback loops that will allow for continuous quality improvement

Delineating this list manages to cycle the discussion back to Principle 1: when establishing an assessment plan from the start, it is vital to understand the purpose of any evaluation pursued. This creates, in a sense, a foundation for "evaluating the evaluation."

Sources and Further Reading

Barbour RS. Checklists for improving rigour in qualitative research: a case of the tail wagging the dog? BMJ. 2001;322(7294):1115–7. http://dx.doi. org/10.1136/bmj.322.7294.1115. Medline:11337448

Barbour RS. The case for combining qualitative and quantitative approaches in health services research. J Health Serv Res Policy. 1999;4(1):39–43. Medline:10345565

Britton A. Evaluating interventions: experimental study designs in health promotion. In: M Thorogood and Y Coombes, editors. *Evaluating Health Promotion.* New York, NY: Oxford University Press; 2010. http://dx.doi.org/10.1093/acprof:oso/9780199569298.003.0004

Brug J, Tak NI, Te Velde SJ. Evaluation of nationwide health promotion campaigns in The Netherlands: an exploration of practices, wishes and opportunities. Health Promot Int. 2011;26(2):244–54. http://dx.doi.org/10.1093/heapro/daq058. Medline:20739324

Crosswaite C, Curtice L. Disseminating research results -- the challenge of bridging the gap between health research and health action. Health Promot Int. 1994;9(4):289–96. http://dx.doi.org/10.1093/heapro/9.4.289.

Goodstadt M, Hyndman B, McQueen DV et al. Evaluation in Health Promotion: Synthesis and Recommendations. *Evaluation in Health Promotion: Principles and Perspectives.* 2001; 517–34.

Israel BA, Cummings KM, Dignan MB, et al. Evaluation of health education programs: current assessment and future directions. Health Educ Q. 1995;22(3):364–89. http://dx.doi.org/10.1177/109019819402200308. Medline:7591790

Jolley GM, Lawless AP, Baum FE, et al. Building an evidence base for community health: a review of the quality of program evaluations. Aust Health Rev. 2007;31(4):603–10. http://dx.doi.org/10.1071/AH070603. Medline:17973619

Plescia M, Groblewski M, Chavis L. A lay health advisor program to promote community capacity and change among change agents. Health Promot Pract. 2008;9(4):434–9. http://dx.doi.org/10.1177/1524839906289670. Medline:17105806

Puska P, Salonen JT, Tuomilehto J, et al. Evaluating community-based preventive cardiovascular programs: problems and experiences from the North Karelia project. J Community Health. 1983;9(1):49–64. http://dx.doi.org/10.1007/BF01318933. Medline:6678258

World Health Organization Regional Publications (Europe). Goodstadt M, Hyndman B, McQueen DV, et al. Evaluation in Health Promotion: Synthesis and Recommendations. *Evaluation in Health Promotion: Principles and Perspectives.* 2001; 517–34.

World Health Organization Regional Publications (Europe). Rootman I, Goodstadt M, Potvin L et al. A Framework for Health Promotion Evaluation. *Evaluation in Health Promotion: Principles and Perspectives.* 2001; 7–38.

13 Conclusion: Sustained Investment in Prevention

We see an integrated state-county rural public health organization – combining the efforts of a supervising health officer and technical staff at the state level with broadly trained public health workers at the county level – as a basis for developing new and continuing services in cooperation with local communities.

– Dr Gordon Macgregor

This quotation from Dr Macgregor was taken from the conclusion to his paper "Social Determinants of Health Practices," published in 1961 as part of a series of reports on the Great Plains Health Study of Colorado. It was one of the first times that the term "social determinants" appears in the academic literature. More pertinently, it represents an early anticipation of a program consistent with community-based prevention educators – 10 years before the launch of the North Karelia Project. This shows that the basic idea has had a long germination, with the following components in view from the beginning:

- Strong public health leadership from the provincial or state level
- Provision of technical support from the centre, allowing field workers to do their job more effectively; presumably this would include developing the evidence base for interventions, risk factor surveillance and other evaluation resources, social marketing campaigns, and possibly a grant program to encourage community efforts
- Professional, population-based field workers with a generalist focus
- Community engagement as a basis for developing or adapting component programs

Figure 13.1. Four Dimensions of CPE Definition.

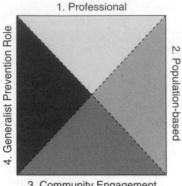

As reviewed below, there is a remarkable overlap between a vision articulated 50 years ago in a western U.S. state and the program that eventually was established through the cancer agency in a western Canadian province.

The community-based prevention educator (CPE) model as found in British Columbia, Canada, was the main occasion and inspiration for this book, so it is appropriate that describing that program occupied the major section of Part A. The following definition was proposed for the CPE-type role that lies at the heart of the British Columbia Cancer Agency's Prevention Programs:

> A professional leader coordinating community-based efforts to reduce the common risk factors and/or progression of cancer and other chronic disease in a defined population.

This definition was elaborated in two different ways in the earlier chapters.

First, a series of rationales were offered for considering a CPE-type program centred on the definition, including the grave burden of cancer and other chronic disease in all jurisdictions of the world, the potential for making progress in prevention by addressing the common risk factors of chronic disease, the usefulness of dividing an entire province into more manageable units within which to pursue population-based prevention efforts, and the various community-based interventions to be coordinated in order to deal comprehensively with intersectoral influences on health. In this way, an argument for CPEs was bound tightly to each of the elements in the CPE definition.

Second, the CPE definition was refined in terms of four constituent dimensions, as follows:

- CPEs are professional leaders rather than volunteers with a limited scope
- CPEs are population-based rather than working within a clinical paradigm
- CPEs work mostly through community engagement rather than program administration
- CPEs are prevention generalists rather than focusing on one intervention or risk factor

This grid is reminiscent of a number of the criteria for effective public health deployment introduced above in the context of Colorado. As summarized in chapter 4, the grid helped to guide the literature search that identified programs in the world comparable to the strategy developed in British Columbia. The checklist approach was important because the actual job titles used in other jurisdictions are quite variable, for example: health promotion officer, cancer control specialist, and extension agent. Ultimately, five jurisdictions (featuring six programs) were identified as suitable to examine across a series of cases studies, including two American states, two European countries, and the Canadian province of Manitoba.

Considering Potential Success Factors

Because they were present in all of the programs by definition, the four dimensions in the previous section were not re-examined as important elements of a CPE-like program. Instead, they were assumed as foundational elements, while several other optional (but important) elements were identified by comparing the case studies with each other and especially with the British Columbia CPE program description. The important elements or principles were described in the preceding three chapters. They represent potential success factors that should at the very least be considered by program planners. The 11 elements are summarized in Figure 13.2.

Figure 13.2. Proposed Success Factors in a CPE-like Program.

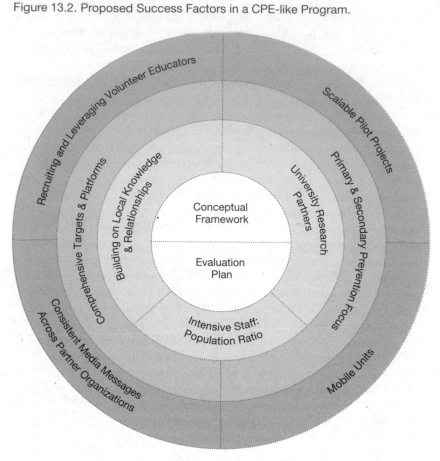

It should be noted that the existence of a theory or conceptual frame-work and a robust evaluation plan are positioned at the core, indicating their relative priority; the rings of other factors are then traced outward in the following order: organizational prerequisites, program targets, and, finally, specific strategies. The sequence moves from the most fun-damental principles, including how – and how many – educators are recruited, to more optional elements, such as the use of lay health ad-visers and mobile prevention units to improve access to services across a jurisdiction.

The key role of a program theory and an evaluation plan has been discussed in detail earlier. Establishing conceptual frameworks and evaluation protocols is challenging because of the intellectual and tangible resources required. It is easy to short-change these elements in a program planning process, but the ensuing prevention educator effort will be weaker as a result. The thinking effort, staff time, and other resources put into developing a solid theoretical foundation and comprehensive evaluation plan will pay dividends. In terms of influencing effectiveness and sustainability, commitment to the twin priorities of theory and evaluation is likely only matched by the basic, ongoing investment in the actual operation of the program itself.

Among different success factors that could be highlighted, a key plank in the foundation of such a program is a commitment to the theory and practice of health promotion, including the various aspects of community engagement that typically have been part of a CPE-like role. Inherent in any program based in health promotion is the challenge of not allowing it to be subsumed in a purely health education mandate. An argument was made in an earlier chapter to the effect that health education may overlap with health promotion but it cannot replace it; in other words, working alongside community partners for the sake of health is not an optional extra but rather a key to sustainable reach into a population. This explains why the CPEs in British Columbia have twin pillars in their role description: community action *and* public education. At the same time, it is important to realize that there is not a complete divorce between the two arenas. By educating a series of larger groups or training individuals who will apply what they have learned to others, CPEs can begin to generate a population-level effect. For instance, in British Columbia, the Tobacco Education and Action Module is delivered to front-line workers such as teachers, counsellors, or social workers, so that the effect of the education becomes multiplied.

The tension between health education and health promotion essentially devolves to the importance of scale. To be effective in the way envisioned in North Karelia, British Columbia, and beyond, the focal unit for a CPE must be bigger than an individual but smaller than a whole province. A CPE must not get caught up in a clinical approach to care, but still have a small enough field of operation to enable ordinary citizens and community groups to band together to make a difference that will actually be felt on the ground – ultimately so that neighbours and organizational partners can take pride in a visible, collaborative achievement.

There is final important element of CPE-like programs that remains to be considered, that is, the investment required to keep such an effort going over the long term. This will be addressed in the next section.

The Importance of Sustained Investment

Given the phenomena of disease latency and the slow onset of chronic disease, it is legitimate to ask whether there is any wisdom in launching a chronic disease prevention strategy without a prior commitment to long-term investment. As implied by the word "chronic," it takes time to see the ultimate outcomes from a prevention program; even intermediate results related to risk factor prevalence do not manifest themselves overnight. This is one reason a prevention program needs to be sustained, so that positive results will have time to emerge and thereby attract resources for further investment. Beyond this mechanism, there is the matter of the process inherent in a CPE-like effort. Health promotion involves multiple activities, some of which are themselves quite time-consuming. One recent textbook on this topic, entitled *Health Promotion Programs: From Theory to Practice*, identified the following activities that require sustained attention: identifying organizational stakeholders; articulating needs, assets, and challenges; building evidence-based component programs; fundraising; advocacy; evaluation; and professional development.

Health promotion work is people intensive, making staff a major expense of prevention programs. Unfortunately, primary prevention is typically the "poor cousin" among the categories of government spending on cancer and other chronic diseases. For example, advocates have pointed out that less than 1% of cancer spending by governments in Canada is dedicated to the primary prevention of cancer. Analysis by the Canadian Cancer Research Alliance (CCRA) has suggested that the picture does not improve very much when spending by the voluntary sector is included: the research budget related to prevention is still less than 2% of total cancer research expenditures. In a recent update, the CCRA reported that 2007 spending on research related to prevention interventions amounted to 1.75% of total cancer research budgets; less than 1% was directed towards understanding interventions dealing with behaviours that influence cancer risk.

There are jurisdictions that do somewhat better, exemplified by the 10% of the Texas Cancer Prevention and Research Institute's budget dedicated to prevention programs and services; in absolute terms, this spending was actually about $22 million for a population about five times that of British Columbia. But even in Texas, it is clear that other aspects of cancer control are still dominant.

With this background on funding, the CPE program may be seen as a means to leverage a relatively modest operating budget dedicated to primary prevention. The CPE model is certainly worth considering as planners attempt to stretch the impact of their limited prevention budgets. A vital challenge involved with such consideration is to assess the level of commitment among policy-makers for sustained investment. It is very counterproductive to "pull the plug" in the middle of an effort where building trust, linkages, and community momentum is essential to the strategy. In short, investment that is not sustained is not a good investment.

To sum up, it is incumbent on policy-makers to be careful in the strategic planning process before launching a prevention educator program, including covering the following elements identified by the Centers for Disease Control and Prevention in the United States:

- identifying program need and capacity,
- planning for resource allocation and use,
- assuring service delivery,
- preparing to respond to critical events, and
- evaluating outcomes.

And even before any other decisions about plans and funding, the level of political will must be assessed. This was the conclusion of the 2007 prevention textbook *The Health Impact of Smoking and Obesity and What to Do about It*, which compared the contemporary challenges of dietary risk factors and physical inactivity with the successful campaigns in the past against smoking:

> The investment of political capital...needs to be maintained. An application of this principle was seen in the Canadian context. When taxation rates on cigarettes were rolled back in the 1990s in response to vigorous lobbying by the tobacco industry, smoking prevalence rates increased dramatically. Sustained courage and political will are basically another type of vital currency to invest in risk factor programs. The battle lines over healthy eating in the developed world are just beginning to be drawn; political capacity needs to be expanded right away to face this challenge.

The finish line in a health care race inevitably leads back to the bottom line. The lesson about sufficient public investment in health promotion and disease prevention, learned the hard way through the ups and downs in the history of tobacco control, must be applied in the same measure to unhealthy eating, inactivity, and obesity. The simple truth is that it is practically useless to devise a multifaceted risk factor plan, announce it to great fanfare, *and then not fund or otherwise support it adequately.*

The Logic of Community-Based Coordination Efforts in Prevention

One of the important health care stories of the present world is that concerns about chronic disease are no longer limited to the higher-income countries. Jurisdictions with far fewer resources than British Columbia, Finland, and North Carolina are looking at pioneers in wealthier settings to see which prevention models might work for them.

The explicit message of this book, anticipated in the two-fold purpose laid out in the introductory chapter, is that policy-makers responding to the burgeoning cases of chronic disease in their jurisdiction ought to strongly consider a CPE-like program to make advances on the prevention front. It also promotes the idea that structuring and implementing such a program ought to be pursued through a careful planning process that involves at least consideration of the success factors identified.

There is a compelling logic to the CPE strategy. First, there is inherent wisdom in the divide-and-conquer approach to prevention coordination, that is, in covering the needs in a province or state in a regionalized way. The advantages are manifold. It is simply easier to conceptualize a smaller, more compact group of people as a target of health improvement; it is easier to travel around and meet with other leaders, local needs can be identified more readily, the existing social connections are more extensive, advertising can be more focused, programs can be tailored, and so on.

Second, as has been seen during the rise of health promotion movements around the world, there is power in coordinating efforts at a community level. It is beyond the scope of this book to trace that history and evidence in detail. However, the North Karelia Project as described herein provides compelling evidence on its own. Over decades of comprehensive community-based efforts, cardiovascular disease and cancer rates have been dramatically reduced in Finland.

It is fair to ask whether there are alternatives to a CPE-like program that could or should be considered. Variations on the community-based prevention approach include the following:

- Primary health care in general, and the specific model known as community-oriented primary care
- Health-promoting hospitals
- Lay health advisers, considered as a stand-alone program
- Formal collaboration of local policy-makers from different social arenas (as, for instance, in the EPODE movement to control childhood obesity, first developed in France and now springing up around the world)

The literature on most of these approaches is vast. To explore each of them in depth would call for a larger tome with a greatly expanded focus. It is important to note that each of these alternative models can actually be integrated in different ways with a CPE strategy; in fact, a complementary program involving lay health advisers has been held up in this book as an important element to consider when planning a CPE-like program. However, most of the other community-based approaches would call for more complex and costly planning and operational phases. Again, in a climate of constrained resources, a community-based prevention educator strategy is an excellent place to start and continue the battle against chronic disease. As has been suggested above, from a global perspective there is no time to lose. The present United Nations Secretary-General, Ban Ki-Moon, recently summed up the urgency in the following way:

> Cancer, diabetes, and heart diseases are no longer the diseases of the wealthy. Today, they hamper the people and the economies of the poorest populations even more than infectious diseases. This represents a public health emergency in slow motion.

Sources and Further Reading

Canadian Cancer Research Alliance. Cancer Research Investment in Canada, 2007. 2009. Available at http://www.ccra-acrc.ca/ (accessed July 2011).

Fertman CI, Allensworth, DD, editors. Health Promotion Programs: From Theory to Practice. Hoboken, New Jersey: Jossey-Bass; 2010.

Krueger H, Williams D, Kaminsky B, et al. *The Health Impact of Smoking and Obesity and What to Do About It*. Toronto: University of Toronto Press; 2007.

MacGregor G. Social determinants of health practices. Am J Public Health Nations Health. 1961;51(11):1709–14. http://dx.doi.org/10.2105/AJPH.51.11.1709. Medline:14467843

Thorogood M, Coombes Y. Conclusions: providing appropriate evidence and influencing policy. In: M Thorogood and Y Coombes, editors. *Evaluating Health Promotion*. New York, NY: Oxford University Press; 2010. http://dx.doi.org/10.1093/acprof:oso/9780199569298.003.0016

Appendix I: Key Informants

International and Canadian Leaders in Comparable Programs

By telephone interview:

Dr Pekka Puska
Director, National Institute for Health and Welfare
Helsinki, Finland

Dr Erkki Vartiainen
Assistant Director, National Institute for Health and Welfare
Helsinki, Finland

Emily Magrath
Health Promotion Manager
Action Cancer, Belfast, Northern Ireland

Debbie Murray
Associate Director, Kentucky HEEL program
Lexington, Kentucky

Debra Armstrong
Director, Kentucky Cancer Program East
Lexington, Kentucky

Kathy Rack
Regional Cancer Control Specialist, Northern Kentucky (Highland
    Heights)
Kentucky Cancer Program

Kim Leathers
Public Health Consultant and CHAP Coordinator
North Carolina Office of Minority Health & Health Disparities, Raleigh, North Carolina

Lynn Watkins
Manitoba Health Promotion Coordinator
Burntwood Regional Health Authority, Thompson, Manitoba, Canada

Kristin Stewart
Clinical Team Supervisor, Community Wellness Team
Interlake Regional Health Authority, Stonewall, Manitoba, Canada

Fiona Jeffries
Health Promotion Education Specialist
Brandon Regional Health Authority, Brandon, Manitoba, Canada

Nancy McPherson
Population Health Planner Analyst
Brandon Regional Health Authority, Brandon, Manitoba, Canada

Betty Kozak
Chronic Disease Prevention Initiative, Training Coordinator
Manitoba Healthy Living, Youth and Seniors
Neepawa, Manitoba, Canada

British Columbia Cancer Agency – Prevention Programs

- Sonia Lamont, Provincial Manager
- El Taylor, Northern Administrator*

CPEs (known in British Columbia as Prevention Educational Leaders)

By survey:

- Wajeeha Raoof, Surrey
- Cory Bendall, Vernon
- Kim Jensen, Kamloops*

- Andrea Winckers, Rossland
- Shirley Baker, Masset
- Sally Errey, Lac la Hache*
- Archie Gaber, Quesnel
- Bill Goodacre, Smithers
- Manon Joice, Fort St John
- Judy Rea, Prince Rupert
- David Sinclair, Terrace
- Lorraine Thibeault, Vanderhoof
- Cheryl Colby, Chilliwack
- Jennifer Leigh, Whistler
- Lori Petryk, Vancouver
- Breann Specht, Vancouver*
- Christy Anderson, Victoria
- Terryl Bertagnolli, Quadra Island*
- John Raven, Gabriola Island

*Followed-up by telephone interview

Appendix II: Cancer Prevention Program Standards in Canada

Table 14.1 Criteria for Bronze Recognition

√	1.	Department with a prevention mandate exists (if combined with secondary prevention / screening, there are dedicated resources / personnel for primary prevention)
√	2.	Primary prevention staff have expertise in public health / health promotion
√	4.	Prevention program is linked or has direct representation on organization's senior executive leadership
√	5.	Organizational vision, mission and philosophies reflect primary prevention goals
√	6.	Primary prevention is included in the cancer agency's business and strategic plans
√	7.	Program has clearly defined goals
√	10.	Program has identified baselines for modifiable risk factors (tobacco, nutrition, etc.) and other indicators (incidence, mortality, etc.)
√	12.	Program takes a population health approach to address existing priorities within the well population
√	13.	Program has short term indicators to assess progress
√	14.	Program interventions are based on best practices or best available evidence
√	16.	Program interventions have an evaluative framework
√	18.	Health education messages are standardized, factual and delivered cost effectively
√	19.	Program provides training and/or continuing education for staff (i.e., professional development)

√   21. Collaborative partnerships for chronic disease prevention in place

√   23. Program engages in knowledge exchange networks to share their findings

√   30. Program partners with non-government organizations

√   33. Program addresses inequities and social determinants of health needs (diversity strategies, aboriginal health, low income population, literacy, etc.)

√   36. Program addresses tobacco control in an appropriate role that adds value

√   37. Program addresses nutrition in an appropriate role that adds value

√   38. Program addresses physical activity in an appropriate role that adds value

√   39. Program addresses sun safety / UVR protection / skin cancer prevention in an appropriate role that adds value

√   40. Program addresses exposure to carcinogens in an appropriate role that adds value

√   42. Program is linked to community level initiatives

√ = current fulfilment by the BCCA Prevention Program

Table 14.2 Criteria for Silver Recognition

√	8.	Primary prevention program role(s) as leader / collaborator / recipient are outlined to maximize resources, avoid duplication, fill gaps
√	28.	Program links with governments to address health policy
√	29.	Program engages communities to create environments that support healthy choices
√	41.	Program collects and disseminates timely, accurate, relevant data about risk factors and programming
√	43.	Program is linked to national cancer prevention initiatives
	11.	Program monitors behavioural risk factors for cancer prevention
	20.	Program provides skill development to communities, partner organizations, other provincial cancer agency staff, etc.
	22.	Collaborative partnerships with cancer treatment and disease management in place
	35.	Program engages clinicians as advocates for primary prevention

√ = current fulfilment by the BCCA Prevention Program

Table 14.3 Criteria for Gold Recognition

√	15.	Program takes a research approach to designing interventions in a way that builds on existing evidence and adds new information to the body of evidence
√	25.	Program utilizes comprehensive school health to reach youth
√	31.	Program partners with other sectors (private sector, education, sports, fashion, transportation, etc.)
	3.	Dedicated budget (within the provincial cancer agency) for primary prevention expressed at least 5% of overall cancer control budget or $5 per capita
	9.	Primary prevention program goals are incorporated into provincial government health plans
	17.	Program utilizes external expert advisory panels to guide programming
	24.	Program accesses or provides grants to build capacity or deliver interventions
	26.	Program provides guidelines for health promotion to clinical care providers
	27.	Program utilizes mass media and best practices in social marketing
	32.	Program addresses continuum of audiences (healthy, at risk, cancer patients and survivors)
	34.	Program includes workplace wellness focus
	44.	Program collaborates with international cancer prevention programs

√ = current fulfilment by the BCCA Prevention Program